Physical Agents Laboratory Manual

Physical Agents Laboratory Manual

Barbara J. Behrens, BS, PTA
Coordinator
Physical Therapist Assistant Program
Mercer County Community College
Trenton, New Jersey

F. A. DAVIS COMPANY • Philadelphia

F. A. Davis Company
1915 Arch Street
Philadelphia, PA 19103

Printed in the United States of America

Last digit indicates print number: 10 9 8 7 6 5 4 3 2 1

Publisher: Jean-François Vilain
Senior Developmental Editor: Crystal Spraggins
Production Editor: Rose Gabbay
Cover Designer: Louis J. Forgione

ISBN Number: 0-8036-0275-8

Preface

Physical agents are techniques or modalities applied to a patient to accomplish a therapeutic treatment goal. They can be wonderful tools to use in conjunction with manual treatment techniques. As clinicians, we strive to improve the quality of life and function for our patients. It is my belief, and the belief of many others, that we can facilitate patient progress through the effective use of physical agent modalities.

This manual requires active participation on the part of the student and the laboratory instructor. There are many potentially right answers to questions raised in the laboratory exercises, and students are encouraged to discuss the rationale for their choices. Instructors are encouraged to listen to the thought processes of students learning to grapple with the intricacies of technology as well as the most complex of all variables, patients.

Keen observation skills are critical to the success of any clinician, so the laboratory exercises in this manual encourage students to observe and record patient responses to the applied interventions. Documentation is also a critical skill in rehabilitation. Therefore, students are instructed to document at least two of the sample patient treatment techniques that were performed during the laboratory activities.

Although it seems obvious to say, common sense is most useful to an individual in a treatment setting. If something sounds inappropriate or does not seem to make sense, it must be challenged. Clinicians need to trust themselves and their instincts. The laboratory activities in the manual invite students to challenge their beliefs and to trust their instincts, fostering the use of commonsense skills. In addition, justification is required for each of the activities that a student might perform in a laboratory exercise. Some of the techniques that are demonstrated in the clinical setting may be different from those presented in the manual. These techniques represent the real world of care, in which there are many options. The common thread is the rationale for the approach taken. If an individual has a sound physiological rationale that is not contraindicated, then the approach selected is probably justified.

Lastly, these laboratory exercises stress the connection between the perceived sensation and the parameter. Students are encouraged to try many of the techniques on themselves so that they can experience what it feels like to be a patient—for example, to have a muscle contract through the use of electrical stimulation. Hopefully, the techniques will be less frightening to students and patients after students have had the opportunity to work through the laboratory exercises.

As an academic, I am always searching for the right books to use with students. That search has led to the development of this laboratory manual. I hope that it meets the needs of other instructors who teach physical agents within their curricula.

Barbara J. Behrens, BS, PTA

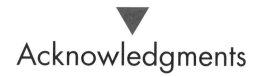

Acknowledgments

As anyone who has ever read book acknowledgments knows, there are many individuals who are involved in the concept, writing, and production of a book.

Without the encouragement of a few close colleagues and friends, JCC, JSM, TES, and SLM, I would never have tackled such an enormous task.

Without the support and patience of my students at Allegheny University of the Health Sciences and Mercer County Community College over the past 5 years, I would not have been able to put a laboratory manual together.

Without the expertise and suggestions of the reviewers, I would not have been able to come up with reasonable case scenarios or patient problems.

Without the gentle but persistent nudging from a "Frenchman" and a "jewel," the project would never have come to fruition.

Without the foundation and work ethic instilled in me by my parents, I would never have been able to focus on the project to see it to completion.

Without Sam, I would not have been able to sit at my desk at home for hours on end, knowing that someone was there with me and loving the fact that my location and activities were known.

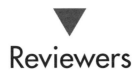

Reviewers

Candace A. Bahner, MS, PT
Director
Physical Therapist Assistant Program
School of Applied Studies
Allied Health Department
Washburn University
Topeka, Kansas

Martha R. Hinman, EdD, PT
Associate Professor
School of Allied Health Sciences
The University of Texas Medical Branch at Galveston
Galveston, Texas

R. Scott Ward, PhD, PT
Assistant Professor
Division of Physical Therapy
University of Utah
Salt Lake City, Utah

J. D. Wendeborn, MS, PT
Coordinator
Physical Therapist Assistant Program
Laredo Community College
Laredo, Texas

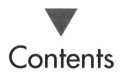

Contents

Therapeutic Heat and Cold
Clinical
Responses

Purpose

Throughout this laboratory exercise, students will be instructed to apply several different forms of thermal agents commonly used in the clinic. The laboratory is designed to emphasize the importance of observational skills and problem solving. It is not designed to outline specific application techniques.

Students are expected to position and drape their patients appropriately, practice safe body mechanics principles, observe patients' responses, and share the responsibility of being both the clinician and the patient.

Objectives

- To familiarize the student with the most common responses to the application of superficial heat and cold (ice, ice packs, iced water)
- To familiarize the student with the importance of skin assessment
- To differentiate between normal and abnormal responses to heat and cold
- To examine skin appearance and document the observations
- To examine responses to heat and cold
- To compare the similarities and differences between the normal responses to heat and cold
- To integrate the problem-solving process for determining techniques for the application of cold to construct accurate descriptions of the sensations associated with the application of heat and cold

Equipment

towels	water basin ice packs	pillow cases
minute timer	thermometer *(high and low*	stethoscope and
ice cubes	*temperatures)*	sphygmomanometer
	hot packs	

Precautions

open wounds	age of the patient
cognitive ability of the patient	metastases
peripheral vascular disease	pregnancy
past experience with the agents used	previous cardiac medical history

Contraindications (H = Heat and C = Cold, unless noted otherwise)

unreliable patient responses	acute inflammation (H)
patients taking anticoagulant	deep vein thrombosis
medications	acute hemmorage (H)
metastases in the treatment area	radiation (x-ray therapy)
decreased sensation in the treatment	existing fever (H)
area to heat, cold, and pain	pregnant uterus during the first
frostbite in the treatment area	trimester of pregnancy
peripheral vascular disease	

LABORATORY EXERCISES

Sensation Comparisons: Superficial Heat and Cold

1. Select two classmate/patients who have different skin types and list them below. Record your observations of their knees in terms of skin type, location of any visible scars [noting the age and condition of the scar(s)], and ability to differentiate between heat and cold, light touch, and dull or sharp pain.

Sensation awareness:

a. Touch the treatment area with your fingertips. Ask the patient to tell you where you are touching him or her, without the patient looking at that area. Ask the patient to describe the sensation.

- Does the patient feel one fingertip or more?

b. Touch the treatment area with something cold, warm, sharp, and blunt.
   - Is the patient able to distinguish between warm and cold?

   - Is the patient able to determine whether he or she was touched by something blunt or sharp?

   - Is the patient able to accurately report a sharp painful sensation (sharp implement)?

Patient 1
Baseline vital signs: _____

Patient 2
Baseline vital signs: _____

2. Position both patients so that they are supine with their knees supported in about 10°–20° of flexion by placing either a towel roll or pillow underneath their knees.
3. Remove two standard-size hot packs from the hydrocollator unit. One hot pack will be applied to each patient. Wrap one hot pack in toweling so that there are four layers of towels between the hot pack and the patient. Wrap the second hot pack in toweling so that there are six layers between the patient and the hot pack. (Use only the towels, not commercial covers, for this exercise.)
4. Record the following information while the hot packs are on your patients' knees:

Patient 1 (four layers of toweling)				
	+3 min	+6 min	+9 min	+12 min
Appearance under the pack				
Patient's report of how the knees feel				
Vital signs				

Patient 2 (six layers of toweling)				
	+3 min	+6 min	+9 min	+12 min
Appearance under the pack				
Patient's report of how the knees feel				
Vital signs				

5. Remove the hot packs from your patients, and observe the knees again, noting any differences between the appearance and sensation that you observed from before the hot pack application. Place the hot packs in the hydrocollator unit for reuse.

6. Ask your patients to get up and walk around. Observe their gait, and ask them to describe how the treated knee feels as they walk on it. Continue to observe the treated area, and determine how long it takes for the knee to return to a pretreatment appearance.

    a. Were there any differences between the perceptions of heat with the two patients? If yes, why do you think this might have occurred? If no, why do you think that this would not have occurred with these two patients?

    b. How would you describe the appearance of your patient's knee after the hot pack had been applied for 6 minutes? (Was there any uniformity to what you observed? Why or why not?)

    c. If your patient had any scars, did the scar tissue respond the same way as the uninvolved tissue?

    d. What would you expect to see if your patient had a recent (4 weeks postoperative) medial meniscectomy scar on the medial aspect of the knee?

    e. What would you expect to see if your patient had a knee replacement 2 years ago?

    f. Which patient from the hot pack application exercise did you expect to feel the heat sooner?

g. Did your expectation happen? Why did or didn't it occur with each of your two patients?

h. How long after you had applied the hot packs did your patients report that the level of heat had reached maximum?

i. What is the normal temperature setting for the hydrocollator unit? (Was the water level in the hydrocollator unit sufficient to cover the hot packs completely? What difference, if any, would the water level make?)

j. In the future, how would you decide whether or not a patient should have four or six layers of towels?

k. Describe how conductive heat sources work. Use terms that your patient will be able to understand.

l. How long would you expect the effects from the hot pack to last? How long did it take for your patients' knees to return to their pretreatment appearance?

m. Based on your patients' responses to questions about how their knees felt when walking after the hot pack application, how, if at all, would this affect your instructions to patients in the future?

n. Did the patients' vital signs change with the application of the hot pack? If yes, how? Why?

Ice Application and Cold Water Immersion

1. Select two classmates/patients who will be having their lateral epicondyle treated with different forms of cryotherapy. One of your patients will be receiving an ice massage directly on the lateral epicondyle, and the other will be immersing his or her elbow in an ice bath. You will be recording your observations of the responses at timed intervals.
   Preparation:
   - Position both patients so that they will be supported and comfortable during the treatment.
   - Wrap an ice cube in a paper towel, or use a prepared "ice pop" for the ice massage.
   - Fill a small basin with about 3 inches of cold water, and pour ice cubes or shaved ice into the water so that the entire surface of the water in the basin is covered with ice. This will serve as the ice bath.
2. Record the following observations:

Ice Massage			
	+3 min	*+6 min*	*+9 min*
Skin appearance			
Patient's report of how the elbow feels			

Ice Bath			
	+3 min	*+6 min*	*+9 min*
Skin appearance			
Patient's report of how the elbow feels			

3. Continue to monitor each patient, noting when he or she feels that the numbness is subsiding and sensation is returning to pretreatment level.
   a. Which patient experienced the most numbness to the treated area? Why?

   b. Which technique was more comfortable for the patient during the treatment itself? What do you think was the reason for this?

   c. In the future, how would you describe the sensations that the patient will feel during the application of ice?

   d. How long did it take for each of your patients to report numbness?

e. How large was the area affected by the treatment for the ice massage? For the ice bath?

f. Was there a relationship between the size of the area affected and the time it took for numbness to occur?

g. How long did the numbness last in each of your patients?

h. How would you describe the appearance of the affected areas 20 minutes after the treatment?

i. When would you choose an ice massage instead of an ice bath?

j. What was the temperature of the ice bath initially? After 20 minutes?

Commercial Ice Packs

Ice packs are available in a variety of sizes and consistencies. Several companies manufacture these packs so that they are readily available for use in both the clinic and the home. Some are intended to be reusable and are therefore covered by a sturdy plastic outer layer. Other commercial cold packs may be composed of chemical compounds contained within a plastic case. Once the compounds mix, they produce a chemical reaction that results in cold temperature production within the pack. Regardless of the type of cold pack used, they rely on conduction as the source of thermal energy exchange. These packs may not be intended for reuse.

You will be applying commercial cold packs in several different manners during this exercise. All of the techniques have their place in the clinic. Whenever there is a variety of techniques for the application of something, it is the responsibility of the clinician to determine the "how" and "why" of the application. There are many potential correct ways of doing something; what is most important is that there is a sound rationale for the choices that are made.

Select three classmates/patients who will be receiving ice packs to their cervical spine and cervical musculature. They should be patients who have demonstrable tightness in their upper trapezius muscles, preferably with palpable nodules in the musculature.

1. Observe their available range of motion (ROM), and record your findings.
2. Palpate the nodules and ask the patients to rate their discomfort on a scale of 1 to 10, where 1 is minimal discomfort and 10 is maximal.
3. Stretch the upper trapezius bilaterally, and note the patient response to the stretch and the ease of movement during the stretch.

PATIENT 1: COMMERCIAL ICE PACK PLACEMENT DIRECTLY ON THE SKIN OF THE PATIENT

Observations

ROM:
Pain scale rating:
Ease of movement:

1. Position your patient so that he or she is supported, the cervical spine is in a neutral position, and the postural muscles are at rest.
2. Remove a cold pack from the freezer, and place it *directly on the upper trapezius* that you observed to be tight and painful for your patient.
3. Cover the area with a towel, and drape your patient. Record the following:

	+3 min	+6 min	+9 min	Longer
Patient's response				
Skin appearance				
Vital signs				

4. Reassess your initial observations.
   ROM:
   Pain scale rating:
   Ease of movement:

PATIENT 2: COMMERCIAL ICE PACK PLACEMENT WITHIN A PILLOWCASE, AND THEN ON THE PATIENT

Observations

ROM:
Pain scale rating:
Ease of movement:

1. Position your patient so that he or she is supported, the cervical spine is in a neutral position, and the postural muscles are at rest.
2. Remove a cold pack from the freezer, and place it in a pillowcase. Apply the covered ice pack to the upper trapezius that you observed to be tight and painful for your patient.
3. Cover the area with a towel, and drape your patient. Record the following:

	+3 min	+6 min	+9 min	Longer
Patient's response				
Skin appearance				
Vital signs				

4. Reassess your initial observations.
   ROM:
   Pain scale rating:
   Ease of movement:

PATIENT 3: COMMERCIAL ICE PACK PLACEMENT WITHIN A DAMP PILLOWCASE, AND THEN ON THE PATIENT

Observations

ROM:
Pain scale rating:
Ease of movement:

1. Position your patient so that he or she is supported, the cervical spine is in a neutral position, and the postural muscles are at rest.
2. Remove a cold pack from the freezer, and place it in a dampened pillowcase. Apply the covered damp pack to the upper trapezius muscle that you observed to be tight and painful for your patient.
3. Cover the area with a towel, and drape your patient. Record the following:

	+3 min	*+6 min*	*+9 min*	*Longer*
Patient's response				
Skin appearance				
Vital signs				

4. Reassess your initial observations.
   ROM:
   Pain scale rating:
   Ease of movement:
   a. Which patients were comfortable with the treatment itself during the ice application? At the end of the treatment?

   b. Which patients reported feeling numbness during the ice application? After how long?

   c. Judging from your pretreatment and treatment observations, which patients responded favorably to the ice pack applications?

   d. Were there any differences in the responses that you observed? If so, what were they?

   e. Which application provided the patient with the least amount of conduction? The greatest?

f. Did your patients respond in some way to each of the techniques employed?

g. What do you think would happen with each of the different techniques? What were you basing your beliefs on? Did they hold true?

h. What would be the rationale for placing a layer of something—either damp or dry—in between the patient and the ice pack?

i. What rationale would there be for *not* placing a layer of something in between the patient and the ice pack? Would there be a difference in outcome between a commercial ice pack and a bag of ice removed from a freezer? If so, what would the difference be?

j. How, if at all, did the sensation vary for the patient between the ice pack, the ice bath, and the ice massage?

k. What would you inform patients that they should feel during the application of any form of cryotherapy?

l. What was the temperature of the cooling unit where the cold packs were stored?

m. Were there any changes in the monitored vital signs? If so, for what reason?

PATIENT SCENARIOS

The following patient scenarios are provided to give you the opportunity to apply some of the theory as well as your experience in the application of superficial heat and cold. You should apply each of the following criteria before deciding to use any of the physical agent modalities. Determine:

- Whether or not cryotherapy is indicated

- When cryotherapy is contraindicated
- If indicated, what your treatment goals(s) should be
- If indicated, *how* cryotherapy should be applied to the patient
- What, if any, are the positioning considerations for the patient
- How you will prepare the patient for what to expect during cryotherapy
- How you will assess whether your selection was appropriate in accomplishing your treatment goal(s)

Case Study A

John has been referred to the physical therapy department for an injury to his left ankle that occurred during a dispute that took place at a hockey game. He is a professional hockey player, and plays goalie. He was playing in the championship game last evening, when another player collided with him on the ice. His left ankle is now edematous, particularly anterior to the lateral malleolus. He has acute tenderness in this area as well. The posterior aspect of the ankle has a large hematoma on both the medial and lateral aspects. There were no fractures noted by the physician who x-rayed the ankle last night. John's chief complaints are pain with palpation and pain with weight bearing as well as an inability to put on his skates because of the edema. John has no significant past medical history. He has previously encountered numerous fractures, sprains, strains, and lacerations during his career.

Case Study B

Marylou is a gymnast who has been referred to the physical therapy department for an injury that she sustained in her cervical spine when she fell from the balance beam during practice this afternoon. She complains of stiffness and pain in the cervical spine with movements in all directions. There were no fractures apparent upon x-ray.

Case Study C

Betty is an elderly woman who has been referred to the physical therapy department for treatment of her osteoarthritic hands. She had an acute exacerbation of her arthritis after canning fresh fruits and vegetables from her garden. She earns her livelihood on the farm where she lives and has rarely seen a medical professional in her lifetime. Betty has diabetes and has lost two toes to frostbite.

Case Study D

George is a perpetual "weekend warrior" who plays softball, soccer, and an occasional touch football game. He has been doing this with his friends on weekends since he graduated from college in 1980. He has been referred to the physical therapy department for an injury to his right knee. He slipped on the grass during a game of "Ultimate Frisbee," and he felt a sharp pain in the medial aspect of his right knee. There were no fractures identified upon x-ray. He is scheduled for a magnetic resonance imaging (MRI) of the knee next week. George complains of instability, pain, and swelling in the knee. He has a history of hypertension, which is being managed by medication.

DOCUMENTATION

The purpose of patient documentation is to provide an accurate record of the treatment that has been rendered. It should contain information about the treatment technique as well as specific details about the application if it had to be performed in a way that was different from the usual manner (e.g., if a patient could not tolerate an ice pack unless it had two layers of cloth, or if an ice bath was effective only if the temperature was 35°F). It should also report the patient's response to the intervention.

For cryotherapy, the documentation must include technique, location, duration, and response.

Select two of the "patients" that you applied modalities to during the laboratory exercise, and write a progress note that includes the patients' subjective complaints, objective information that you recorded, the physical agent that was applied, manner of application, response to the applied physical agent, and your assessment.

Laboratory Questions

1. After application of one of the forms of cryotherapy, how would the skin that had been treated appear?

2. After application of a hot pack, how would the skin that had been treated appear?

3. How would you be able to tell which modality had been applied to a patient—heat or cold?

4. During the first section of the laboratory exercises, you were instructed to observe the skin for scars or any other abnormalities. How would the presence of a scar in the treatment area potentially affect your treatment?

5. Does the age of a scar have any significance?

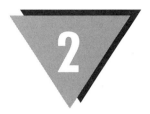

Clinical Application Techniques for Therapeutic Heat

Purpose

This laboratory exercise involves clinical application techniques for a wide variety of therapeutic heating agents, including hydrocollator packs, paraffin, Fluidotherapy, and short-wave diathermy. Students are expected to receive and administer treatments to their classmates and to record observations from both perspectives, where indicated.

The exercises are intended to allow students to compare different application techniques, determine alternative treatment setups, learn to describe and document the sensations of different forms of therapeutic heat, and begin to familiarize themselves with the similarities and differences of the heating agents.

Objectives

- To provide the student with a variety of sensory experiences in response to the application of several forms of therapeutic heating agents, including hydrocollator packs, paraffin, Fluidotherapy, and short-wave diathermy
- To provide the student with practical application challenges for thermal agents
- To provide the student with opportunities to compare and contrast different forms of therapeutic heat
- To initiate the problem-solving process for determining appropriate application techniques for therapeutic heat

Equipment

towels	minute timer	paraffin unit
gowns	hydrocollator packs	short-wave diathermy
pillows (and cases)	(various sizes)	thermometer
plastic bags	Fluidotherapy	

Precautions

open wounds

cognitive ability of the patient

pregnancy

peripheral vascular disease

advanced age

previous experience with the physical
agents

operation of a mechanical traction unit
or electrical stimulation unit
(within 10 feet of a diathermy unit
that is running)

Contraindications

pregnancy (during the first trimester
for *all* thermal agents if applied in
the low back or over the uterus)

undressed or infected wounds

presence of a pacemaker

metastasis

lack of sensation in the treatment area

Diathermy is specifically contraindicated in the presence of metal implants, stimulation devices, or jewelry; over a pregnant uterus; over the eyes; over the gonads, over edematous areas; for the treatment of rheumatoid arthritic joints; and without a towel on the surface of the skin. In addition, diathermy devices should not be operated within close proximity of other individuals who might be pregnant or have implanted stimulation devices.

LABORATORY EXERCISES

Hydrocollator Packs (Hot Packs)

Select three classmates/patients who will have hot packs applied to their lower backs. You will be positioning them differently to compare the conduction of thermal energy from the hot pack to each of the patients. As with all treatments, inspect the area and note the presence of scars, edema, muscle guarding, or impairments in sensation.

1. Position one patient prone with a pillow underneath the abdomen and ankles to reduce lordosis and permit treatment in a neutral spine position.

    Remove a standard-size hot pack, and place it in a commercial cover. Place a folded towel over the treatment area, and place the hot pack on top of the folded towel. Drape your patient.

    a. Ask the patient to describe how the hot pack feels on his or her back.

   b. Ask the patient to describe the sensation after:
     5 minutes:

     8 minutes:

     10 minutes:

   c. Does your patient ever report that the hot pack is getting too warm? If yes, after how long, and what did you do to provide relief?

2. Position your patient so that he or she is supine, with a pillow underneath the head and knees for support. Clothing should be removed in the treatment area so that it is not in the way of the hot pack.

    Remove a standard-size hot pack, and place it in a commercial cover. Place a folded towel on top of the cover, and ask your patient to lift himself or herself up so that you can place the hot pack underneath.

   a. Ask the patient to describe how the hot pack feels on his or her back.

   b. Ask the patient to describe the sensation after:
     5 minutes:

     8 minutes:

     10 minutes:

   c. Does the patient ever report that the hot pack is getting too warm? If yes, after how long, and what did you do to provide relief?

3. Position your patient so that he or she is side lying. You will need to adjust the patient's position to ensure that the hot pack is in good contact with the lumbar spine. It is important that the patient be well supported in the neutral position and is comfortable. (A wall or strap may work well.) Describe the position that you decided on, and indicate the rationale for your choice.

Remove a standard-size hot pack, and place it in a commercial cover. Place a folded towel over the treatment area, and place the hot pack on the folded towel. Secure the hot pack in place.

a. Ask the patient to describe how the hot pack feels on his or her back.

feels good

b. Ask the patient to describe how the hot pack feels after:
   5 minutes:

feels good; could be warmer

warmest 8 minutes:

warmer now; but still feels good.

   10 minutes:

about the same; not too hot

c. Does the patient ever report that the hot pack is getting too warm? If yes, after how long, and what did you do to provide relief?

No

Remove the hot packs from your patients after 15 minutes, and reassess the treatment area. Leave a layer of toweling on the treatment area while you return the hot pack to the hydrocollator unit.

4. Subjectively, which patient felt the most comfortable initially?

all felt good

5. Were all three patients still comfortable after 10 minutes? If not, which one wasn't? What would your explanation be for this?

Supine- too hot after 10 min.
B/c of pressure of body wt.

6. How long did it take for the heat from the hot pack to reach maximum temperature with each of the patients?

Prone:_____ Supine: _8 min._ Side lying:_____

Added 1 towel.

Is this what you expected? Why or why not?

Yes; B/c the weight of one's body is going to make it the heat more intense.

7. Which position made it easiest for you to add more towel layers?

Prone

8. Which patient had the greatest amount of erythema after hot pack removal? Why?

Supine, the pressure of his body was greatest making

9. Which patient had the least amount of erythema after hot pack removal? Why?

Side-lying; hot-pack not close to body

10. When would each of the positions that you tried be indicated (prone, supine, and side lying?

Side lying - pregnancy

11. How long after hot pack removal did it take for the appearance of the treated area to return to its pretreatment coloring?

after 5 min. Supine & prone still had redness.

12. There are a variety of sizes and shapes of hot packs to allow for better contouring and therefore conduction of the thermal energy of the hot pack. Try them and see what size or shape works best in the following areas of the body. Describe your patient positioning techniques.

a. Shoulder:

b. Hip:

c. Knee:

d. Cervical spine:

Paraffin

Select two classmates/patients who will have paraffin applied to their hands. You should inspect and wash their hands, recording any observations you make. Paraffin can be applied in several different methods. For this exercise, you will be comparing the dip method to the continuous immersion method.

1. What is the temperature of the paraffin unit that you will be using? Is this considered hot? Appropriate? Is this the same temperature that has been used in the other paraffin units within the lab?

2. Which method would you expect to provide the most vigorous form of heat? Why?

DIP METHOD

1. Ask your patient to dip his or her hand and wrist into the paraffin unit, remove it, and let the paraffin harden. Then instruct the patient to redip for 8 to 10 layers of paraffin.
2. Wrap the dipped hand in plastic wrap and then in a towel.
3. Position your patient for a 15-minute treatment time.
   a. How does the paraffin feel to your patient?
   Initially:

   After 3 minutes:

   After 6 minutes:

   After 9 minutes:

   After 12 minutes:

  b. Ask your patient to describe how his or her hand feels after the paraffin is removed and returned to the parafifin unit to be remelted.

4. Reassess your patient, and document your observations.

CONTINUOUS IMMERSION

1. Ask your patient to immerse his or her hand and wrist in the paraffin unit, remove it, and let the paraffin harden. Then ask the patient to reimmerse the hand and wrist in the unit and leave it in the unit. The patient should be careful to not move the fingers or break the "glove" of paraffin that had initially formed.
2. Position your patient so that he or she is comfortable and will continue to be comfortable and supported during a 15-minute treatment time for immersion in the unit.
  a. How does the paraffin feel to your patient?
    Initially:

    After 3 minutes:

    After 6 minutes:

    After 9 minutes:

    After 12 minutes:

  b. Was your patient able to withstand the full treatment time in the paraffin unit?

    Which patients may not be able to withstand the entire time? Why?

c. Ask your patient to describe how the hand feels after it is removed from the unit, and remove the paraffin from the hand. Return the paraffin to the unit to be remelted.

3. Reassess your patient, and document your observations.

   a. Which technique was "tolerated better" by the patient? Why?

4. Describe the appearance of each of the treated hands after removal from the paraffin. Is there a difference? Why or why wouldn't you expect to see one?

5. What types of patients would be good candidates for each of the techniques and why?

6. What would you do if, prior to immersing your patient in the paraffin unit, you noted that the temperature was 140°F?

Fluidotherapy

Select two classmates/patients who will be immersing one of their hands into a Fluidotherapy unit. Inspect and wash their hands, recording any additional observations that you make. You will be comparing two different treatment techniques, one that is used to help promote the healing of uninfected wounds and the other that is used to provide heat and desensitization to the immersed part.

1. What is the temperature of the Fluidotherapy unit?
2. What is the desired treatment temperature?
3. What could you do to ensure that the unit was the right temperature when you needed it?

"BAGGED" OR "GLOVED" TECHNIQUE

1. After washing and drying your patient's hand, secure either a plastic bag or glove so that it is "airtight." Tape the bag or glove so that the edges are covered with tape that is adhered to the skin. It may be necessary to use two plastic bags if they are thin.
2. Place the bagged hand into the media in the unit, and secure the port around the forearm.
3. Position your patient so that he or she will be supported and comfortable for the next 10 to 12 minutes.
4. Turn the unit on without any turbulence or agitation. Then adjust the turbulence so that it is comfortable for the patient.
   a. Ask your patient to describe how his or her hand feels:
      Initially:

      After 3 minutes:

      After 6 minutes:

      After 9 minutes:

      After 12 minutes:

   b. Does it feel dry or damp? Does that sensation change? If yes, when?

   c. Does he or she report any desire to "move" in the media? Can he or she?

5. Turn off the unit, slowly remove the patient's hand from the unit, and carefully brush the media back into the port. Remove the bag or glove. Secure the port and reassess your patient, documenting your observations.

a. What is the temperature of the unit after the treatment time?

UN-"BAGGED" TECHNIQUE

1. After washing and drying the hand that will be immersed in the Fluidotherapy unit, instruct your patient to reach into the media with his or her hand. Secure the sleeve of the unit so that no media will escape during the treatment time.
2. Position your patient so that he or she will be supported and comfortable for the 12-minute treatment time.
3. Turn the unit on without any agitation. Gradually adjust the agitation so that the patient is comfortable.
   a. Ask your patient to describe how his or her hand feels.
      Initially:

      After 3 minutes:

      After 6 minutes:

      After 9 minutes:

      After 12 minutes:

   b. Does it feel dry or damp? Does this sensation change? If yes, after how long?

   c. Does your patient express any desire to move in the media? Can he or she?

4. Turn the unit off, slowly remove the hand from the unit, and brush the media back into the port. Secure the port and reassess your patient, documenting your observations.

a. What is the temperature of the unit after the treatment time?

b. How do the descriptions of the treatment technique sensations vary between your two patients? Why do you think that this is true?

c. How would you describe the sensations that a patient will experience in a Fluidotherapy unit?

d. Was there any great difference ($\pm$ 5°) between the pre-treatment temperature and the post-treatment temperature of the unit? Why or why not?

e. When would the use of a glove or bag on the treatment area be indicated?

f. What about the treatment is "lost" when a glove is worn by the patient during treatment? What is gained?

g. Describe the rationale for the positioning of the ports on the unit.

h. What would be the indications for treatment with Fluidotherapy?

Short-Wave Diathermy

Short-wave diathermy is a treatment modality that has been used for many years owing to its ability to elevate internal tissue temperatures in relatively large treatment areas and selectively heating muscle tissue, without placing anything but a towel on the surface of the skin. Because of the increased number of precautions associated with this technique, clinicians have not always used the modality in situations where it may be appropriate. Recent research has yielded further support for the use of diathermy as both a thermal and nonthermal treatment modality.

Diathermy units may have a variety of applicators available for use. Treatment drum applicators are applied in pairs and may be placed parallel to each other on opposite sides of a joint. This technique allows for penetration through the joint, focusing on two primary joint surfaces, such as the medial and lateral aspects. Treatment drums may also be used to encompass a larger area by placing one drum proximally and one drum distally on the same surface of the treatment area. This technique may enhance the conduction through larger, more longitudinally oriented structures.

Some diathermy units have treatment cables that can be used to encase the treatment area. These treatment cables have spacer bars that maintain an equal distance between the individual cables themselves. The cables would be wrapped around an extremity (over the toweling that is on the surface of the skin). This form of applicator would allow for treatment to all joint surfaces rather than just medial and lateral aspects of a joint, as would be treated with drum applicators.

This exercise focuses on the thermal application techniques for diathermy and the sensations that are common with this application. Nonthermal application techniques would use the same principles for setup, but there would be no reported sensation from the patient.

1. Select one classmate/patient who will have continuous thermal short-wave diathermy applied to the medial aspect of the knee. Inspect the area, and document your observations.

2. Position your patient so that they will be supported and comfortable for the 15-minute treatment time. (Determine how to apply the applicators that you have available to you.)

3. Drape the knee with a towel so that the towel is in contact with the skin.

4. Familiarize yourself with all of the controls of the unit:
   - Treatment timer
   - Intensity control
   - Tuning capability

5. Position the treatment applicator(s) (drum, plates, or cables). How did you decide to position your patient? Why? Which applicator did you decide to use and what was your rationale for your selection?

6. Turn the unit ON. Gradually increase the intensity until the patient begins to feel something.
   a. Ask your patient to describe how the knee feels:
   Initially:

   After 3 minutes:

   After 6 minutes:

After 9 minutes:

After 12 minutes:

    b. Did your patient perspire at all during the treatment time? If yes, what did you do?

7. Turn the unit OFF. Remove the treatment applicator(s). Unplug the unit from the wall outlet.
8. Reassess your patient, and document your observations.

    a. How, if at all, did the appearance of the knee change during the treatment time?

    b. How would the sensations reported by the patient be different if you were treating the hip? The thigh? The back? Why?

    c. What potential advantages are there for thermal treatments with diathermy?

    d. What types of patients do you think would benefit from thermal treatments with diathermy? What is your rationale for your choices?

e. Did the diathermy produce the type of sensations that you expected it to?

f. How would you explain this form of treatment to a patient in the future?

PATIENT SCENARIOS

Read through the patient scenarios, and determine the following:
- Which of the forms of therapeutic heat would be indicated. Provide your rationale.
- What application technique(s) you would employ. (If there is more than one option, describe each.)
- When heat would be contraindicated.
- What precautions there are for each patient.
- What additional information if any, would you need to know prior to applying therapeutic heat to each patient.
- How you will assess whether or not your selection was appropriate and accomplished the stated treatment goals.
- How you would position the patient for treatment.

Case Study A

Richard is a 55-year-old retired truck driver who has been referred to the physical therapy department for treatment to relieve pain and stiffness in his right knee. X-rays revealed arthritic changes in both knees. He had a medial meniscectomy in the right knee 2 years ago. His recent complaints of pain and stiffness are related to his present leisure and work activities. Richard is an avid golfer, a country and western dancer, and a chauffeur.

Case Study B

Charlotte is a 50-year-old secretary who has been referred to the physical therapy department for treatment to relieve symptoms associated with the automobile accident that she was involved in 3 weeks ago. She is having difficulty maintaining an upright position because of severe headaches, back pain, and intermittent paresthesias in her dominant right hand. She is a small-framed woman, who taught aerobics classes 5 nights a week. She is unable to teach at all now. There were no fractures, and she is otherwise healthy.

Case Study C

Mike is a 37-year-old carpenter who has been referred to the physical therapy department subsequent to a fall that took place while he was working. He fell from a second-story scaffolding in a house that he was working on. In an attempt to break his fall, he reached for a nearby ladder and landed on a cement-slab floor. His chief complaints are of pain with internal rotation, abduction, and horizontal adduction of the right shoulder. He has marked muscle guarding in the paraspinal musculature bilaterally throughout the lumbar spine. He also reinjured his left ankle, which he has sprained approximately seven times before. As an independent contractor, he is anxious to resume work as quickly as possible to keep the project on schedule. Other than the injuries noted, he had no significant medical history. His prior experiences with physical therapy yielded unsuccessful results with ultrasound.

Case Study D

Jimmy is a 67-year-old retired factory worker who has been referred to the physical therapy department to help relieve chronic arthritic joint stiffness and pain in his hands. He has diabetes, and he has had a below-the-knee amputation on the right leg and ambulates with a prosthesis and no assistance device. He is an active man who is now frustrated by his inability to work on his sailboat. He cannot tie the lines without pain, and he thinks that the lines are therefore insecure.

DOCUMENTATION

For the treatment to be reproduced by another clinician or reviewed by another individual who was not present, documentation must include the following:
- Treatment modality used, such as hot packs, paraffin, Fluidotherapy, and diathermy
- Area(s) treated, including which aspect of that area (e.g., medial knee, lateral knee, anterior posterior and lateral hip)
- How long the treatment with the modality lasted (5 minutes, 20 minutes, etc.)
- Treatment positioning, *only* if it was unusual (side lying, seated, etc.)
- Assessment and reassessment by the clinician with objective measures, such as pain scales, ROM, strength, and so forth.

Select two of the "patients" that you applied modalities to during the laboratory exercise, and write a progress note that includes the patient's subjective complaints, objective information that you recorded, the physical agent that was applied, manner of application, response to the applied physical agent, and your assessment.

LABORATORY QUESTIONS

1. Which of the therapeutic heating agents became progressively warmer during the treatment time?

2. Which of the therapeutic heating agents maintained a constant amount of heat during the treatment time?

3. Which of the therapeutic heating agents cooled off quickly after application?

4. Which of the therapeutic heating agents would be most applicable for conditions involving the hands and feet?

5. If your patient could not tolerate a prone position during the application of therapeutic heat to relieve paraspinal muscle guarding for treatment to his or her lower back, what alternative(s) do you have?

6. Which of the therapeutic heat modalities would be contraindicated for a patient who has had joint replacement surgery?

7. List two treatment alternatives for therapeutic heat application for a patient who has had joint replacement surgery.

8. What additional considerations would there be for positioning a patient so that the area being treated was on top of a hot pack? Is this a viable treatment option?

9. Describe the difference(s) in sensation that a patient will feel between paraffin (dip) and hot pack application.

10. Describe the difference(s) in sensation that a patient will feel between hot packs and diathermy application.

11. Describe the difference(s) in sensation that a patient will feel between paraffin and Fluidotherapy application techniques.

Clinical Application Considerations and Techniques for Therapeutic Ultrasound

Purpose

Ultrasound is one of the most common physical agents used in the clinic today. There are numerous manufacturers of ultrasound devices, and there are a wide variety of parameters available on these devices. Technological advances have offered new options for treatment. Consequently, it becomes increasingly more important for clinicians to understand not only the indications, precautions, and contraindications for ultrasound, but also the meaning of some of the technology and its impact on what they do with ultrasound.

This laboratory exercise starts by familiarizing students with the devices themselves. Students are guided through the identification of the available parameters that they have to observe. They are guided through a testing procedure to familiarize them with both the beam output and some of the terminology regarding the acoustical energy beam. Laboratory exercises are then focused on the clinical application of the previously identified parameters and the patients' responses to the application of the parameters.

Students are expected to be both the "patient" and the clinician so that they practice applying ultrasound and experience the treatment itself. A variety of parameters will be used, compared, and contrasted. Students are expected to be able to recognize appropriate parameters for the accomplishment of a specific treatment goal and to be able to provide a rationale for their selections.

Objectives

- To familiarize the student with the available parameters of therapeutic ultrasound devices
- To provide the student with the opportunity to apply and receive therapeutic ultrasound
- To provide the student with practical application challenges for ultrasound and the decisions that need to be made regarding patient positioning, parameter selection, and device selection (based on available parameters)
- To strengthen the importance of assessment techniques and their application both prior to and following the application of ultrasound
- To provide the student with the opportunity to contrast and compare patients' responses to the application of different parameter sets

Equipment

variable frequency ultrasound unit (1 MHz, 3 MHz)	towels
	pillows
various sizes of transducers	cellophane tape
ultrasound gel (acoustically conductive gel)	cup of water

Precautions

open wounds	age of the patient
cognitive ability of the patient	previous experience with ultrasound
pregnancy	metal implants
peripheral vascular disease	artificial joints

Contraindications

over a pregnant uterus	with undiagnosed painful conditions	with abscesses
over a metastasis	over orbits of the eyes	over a pacemaker
with thermal application over an insensate area	directly over the gonads	over psoriasis
with tuberculosis	over a thrombus or with thrombophlebitis	over epiphysis of growing bone

LABORATORY EXERCISES

Orientation to the Ultrasound Equipment

1. Select an ultrasound unit, and record the following information:
   a. Manufacturer:
   b. Last inspection date or manufacture date:

   c. Available frequencies:
   d. Available transducer sizes:
   e. Effective radiating areas (ERAs):
   f. Available duty cycles:
   g. Beam nonuniformity ratios (BNRs):
2. Locate each of the following, and inspect them for wear:
   a. Generator
   b. Coaxial cable
   c. Transducer
   d. Timer
   e. Intensity control
   f. Duty cycle control

Testing the transducer for acoustical output:
3. Select a transducer that is waterproof, and make a tape ring around the transducer, so that you are creating a "well" that can be filled with water. (Consult instruction manual to determine whether or not the transducer is waterproof.) Pour some tap water into the well so that the water depth is about ¼ inch deep. Set the following parameters: 1 MHz, continuous wave (CW) at an intensity of 1.5 W/cm².
4. Look at the transducer surface.
   a. Is there a disturbance in the water? If yes, then there is acoustical output from the transducer.
   b. What would *no* disturbance in the surface of the water indicate?

Understanding specifications and their meaning: ERA and BNR:
5. Look down at the transducer surface from the top, and note how much of the surface of the transducer is producing disturbances in the water. This is like looking at the ERA of the transducer. Observe the disturbance to see whether it is a high percentage or low percentage of the surface area.
6. Set the intensity to 1 W/cm². Look at the intensity indicator on the unit that you are using. If you can, select power output. Power is an indication of the energy being delivered by the transducer in total. Some units have an analog meter with two scales on it, one is intensity measured in watts/cm² and the other is power measured in watts. Other units have a switch or button that would shift the reading to either power or intensity.
   a. What does the power reading now indicate?

   b. What is the ERA of the transducer that you are testing? (Intensity in watts/cm² × ERA in cm² = power in watts.)

7. Look at the surface of the water through the tape from the side. Gently move the water around so that you can see a cross-section of the acoustical energy leaving the transducer. This is like looking at the BNR of the transducer. You are looking for a uniformity to the beam. Lower BNRs are represented by few peaks and valleys. Higher BNRs are represented by many peaks and valleys and many irregularities to the beam of energy.

8. Repeat these steps with another frequency, other pulsed duty factors (DFs), and other transducers that are available.

3 MHz	10 cm² head	Other sizes:
50% duty factor	7.5 cm² head	Other duty factors:
20% duty factor	5 cm² head	

Treatment Techniques

APPLICATION OF ULTRASOUND TO SHOULDER

1. Select a classmate/patient who will have his or her shoulder treated with ultrasound. Determine what parameters you would use and your rationale for their selection if the patient had a chronic supraspinatus tendinitis. The patient was referred for physical therapy to assist in decreasing joint pain, stiffness, and increasing ROM, which is limited because of pain.
   a. Describe the parameters you selected and the rationale for each selection.
      - Frequency:

      - Intensity:

      - Transducer size:

      - DF:

      - Treatment time:

2. Determine how you will be positioned and how your patient will be positioned so that the treatment technique can be optimized.
   a. Describe your choices and your rationale.

   b. What should your patient feel during the treatment?

   c. What assessments will you make prior to treatment?

d. Explain the treatment and anticipated effects to your patient. Use language that your patient, not a classmate, would understand.

3. Treat your patient using the parameters that you have selected.
   a. How quickly should you move the transducer?

   b. What is your patient's response to the ultrasound?

   c. How long after you initiated treatment with the ultrasound did sensation, if any sensation, occur from the ultrasound?

   d. Reassess your patient's response to treatment, and document your observations.

APPLICATION OF ULTRASOUND TO KNEE

1. Select a classmate/patient who will have his or her knee treated with ultrasound. Assume that the patient had an arthroscopic medial meniscectomy approximately 4 weeks ago. The patient is complaining of pain at the superior medial border of the patella. ROM is limited to 10°–50°, and passive flexion beyond 90° produces stretching pain in the quadriceps.
   a. Determine what your treatment area(s) will be, what you will be treating, and why.

   c. What parameters will you use?

   d. What position(s) will you treat your patient in?

   e. What assessment tools will you use pretreatment?

   f. What sensation if any, should the patient feel during treatment?

   g. If the patient does feel a sensation, where would you expect it to be felt: superficial or deep?

   h. What would your options be to reduce an adverse sensation?

2. Treat your patient, and record his or her response to the treatment.

NONTHERMAL, MECHANICAL, AND THERMAL EFFECTS OF ULTRASOUND

1. Identify four classmates/patients who have palpable fibrocystic nodules in the upper trapezius that are painful to palpation. You will be comparing various ultrasound treatment parameter sets and reporting your results to your classmates and laboratory faculty.
2. Position and drape the patients so that they are comfortably supported and the upper trapezius is at rest. (All patients should be positioned identically for this exercise.)
3. Perform the following:
   Palpate the upper trapezius and ask your patient to rate the degree of discomfort that he or she experiences during palpation, recording it on a scale of 1 to 10.

   Patient 1 pain rating:
   Before treatment ____/10   *After treatment* ____/10
   Parameters: 3 MHz, 50% DF, 0.5 W/cm^2 for 2 minutes. Limit the treatment area to the nodule that was palpated.
   a. What should the patient feel during the treatment?

   Repalpate the area after treatment, and record the pain rating and any change that you perceived from when you initially palpated the area.

   Palpate the upper trapezius, and ask your patient to rate the discomfort that he or she experiences during the palpation, recording it on a scale of 1 to 10.

   Patient 2 pain rating:
   Before treatment ____/10   *After treatment* ____/10
   Parameters: 3 MHz, 50% DF, 0.5 W/cm^2 for 5–8 minutes depending on the transducer size (2 minutes per treatment area equal to the size of the transducer). Insonate the entire trapezius.
   b. What should the patient feel during the treatment?

   Repalpate the area after the time is up, and reassess the level of discomfort that your patient experiences with palpation. Record your observations regarding how the area feels to you, and record the patient's response.

Palpate the upper trapezius, and ask your patient to rate the discomfort that he or she experiences during the palpation, recording it on a scale of 1 to 10.

Patient 3 pain rating:
Before treatment   _____/10   *After treatment*   _____/10
Parameters: 1 MHz, CW, 1.5 W/cm², and sonate the entire trapezius for 8 minutes.
c. What should the patient feel during the treatment?

Repalpate the area after the time is up, and reassess the level of discomfort that your patient experiences with palpation. Record how the area feels to you and the patient's response.

Palpate the upper trapezius and ask your patient to rate the discomfort that he or she experiences during the palpation, recording it on a scale of 1 to 10.

Patient 4 pain rating:
Before treatment   _____/10   *After treatment*   _____/10
Parameters: 1 MHz, CW, 1.5 W/cm², and sonate just the palpable nodule for 2 minutes.
d. What should the patient feel during the treatment?

Repalpate the area after the time is up, and reassess the level of discomfort that your patient experiences with palpation. Record how the area feels to you, and the patient's response.

e. Which of these parameter sets produced palpable differences in the upper trapezius?

e. Why do you believe that you saw the results that you observed?

f. When would 3 MHz be more appropriate than 1 MHz?

g. When would pulsed ultrasound be more appropriate than continuous ultrasound?

h. When would treating the nodule instead of treating the entire muscle be indicated?

i. If you only had a 1-MHz unit and the area that you were treating would be better suited for 3 MHz, what would you do? (Which of the parameters might you expect to have to adjust?)

j. Were there any differences in the sensation perceived by the patient during the treatment with the various parameter sets? (Did you have to adjust any of the parameters. If yes, which ones, and why?)

PATIENT SCENARIOS

Read through the patient scenarios, and determine the following: (If you feel that you need more information regarding the patient, consult your instructor for clarification.)
- Which of the parameter sets for therapeutic ultrasound would be indicated (provide your rationale)
- What application technique you would employ
- When ultrasound would be contraindicated
- What precautions there are for the patient described
- What additional information if any, you would need to know prior to applying therapeutic ultrasound to the patient described
- How you will assess whether or not your selection was appropriate in accomplishing the stated treatment goals
- How you would position the patient for treatment

Case Study A

Betty is a 55-year-old manager of a multimedia theater who has been referred to the physical therapy department for treatment to relieve pain and muscle guarding in her cervical spine. She has a prior history that includes osteoarthritis, three cervical strains, and a laminectomy and fusion of C5 and C6, which was performed approximately 15 years ago.

Case Study B

Cindy is a 50-year-old amateur speed trial race car driver who has been referred to the physical therapy department for lower back pain and muscle guarding that she noticed after racing last weekend. The pain radiates into the buttocks and down to the left popliteal space. She has a history of lower back strains due to lifting injuries while working as a roofer when she was younger. She is 5 feet tall and weighs 90 pounds. Traction relieves her radiating pain, but heat relieves her muscle guarding.

Case Study C

Phil is a 40-year-old package delivery service driver who has been referred to the physical therapy department subsequent to intermittent pain, weakness, and cramping in his dominant left-hand thumb. Extension and abduction of the thumb reproduce his pain. There are no fractures, and he describes the onset of the pain as gradual. The hand is edematous with exquisite tenderness over the anatomical "snuffbox."

Case Study D

Jim is a 32-year-old police officer who has been referred to the physical therapy department for treatment of his right forearm. He was involved in an automobile accident 6 weeks ago during which his vehicle collided head on with another vehicle. He had multiple fractures and contusions that have now healed. His chief complaint centers on his wrist and forearm, which were fractured and pinned with a steel plate between the distal radius and ulna. He has pain with stretching of the supinators into pronation. His incision is well healed, and he has normal sensation in the upper extremity.

DOCUMENTATION

For the treatment to be reproduced by another clinician or to be reviewed by another individual who was not present, documentation must include the following:
- Parameters of the treatment
- Frequency of the ultrasound administered
- DF
- Intensity
- Treatment area
- Treatment time

(The treatment time is related to the size of the transducer used, so it is not imperative that this be recorded. However, specific facilities or insurance carriers may require this information in patient documentation.)

It is also not important for the medium used to be recorded, unless it is something other than ultrasound gel or lotion.

Position for treatment is determined by the treatment goals. The only time the position must be recorded is if it is unusual. If stretching is taking place during the ultrasound administration, then the position and the type of stretch need to be recorded.

Assessment and reassessment tools must be recorded in the patient record.

Select two of the "patients" that you applied modalities to during the laboratory exercise, and write a progress note that includes the patient's subjective complaints, objective information that you recorded, the physical agent that was applied, manner of application, the response to the applied physical agent, and your assessment.

LABORATORY QUESTIONS

1. How might knowledge of a high BNR alter the application of ultrasound?

2. How might knowledge of a low BNR alter the application of ultrasound?

3. How would the knowledge of the ERA of a unit potentially benefit the clinician?

4. What tissue types absorb the greatest amount of acoustical energy?

5. Where will a patient first report a sensation from ultrasound?

6. Using terminology that a patient would understand, describe how ultrasound works, and why they don't hear it and may not feel it.

7. If your were directed to treat an area with ultrasound that was larger than 2 times the size of the transducer, and the goal was to produce heat, what would be the most appropriate action to take? Why?

8. What difference would it make if the coupling media were not acoustically conductive?

9. If a pharmacist "whipped up" a phonophoretic medication for use in the physical therapy department, what would you need to know about the mixture? Why?

10. Outline the steps necessary for a successful treatment with phonophoresis.

Electrical Stimulation Parameters, Responses, and Sensations

Introduction to Direct Current Application Techniques

Purpose

This laboratory exercise is designed to familiarize students with the common terminology for electrical stimulation devices. There are a wide variety of adjustable parameters and often several names for the same parameter. Students will be guided through a familiarization process with the devices, and then they will be applying electrodes to each other and adjusting individual parameters. This laboratory is not intended to demonstrate specific electrode placement sites for the accomplishment of therapeutic goals; rather, it is an informal practice session intended to foster a minimum comfort level with electrical stimulation devices.

The later portion of the laboratory focuses on the application of DC for iontophoresis. Students will be "phoresing" tap water across the skin and noting changes that occur.

Objectives

- To familiarize the student with the available parameters of electrical stimulation devices

- To provide the student with the opportunity to discover the relationships between technical terminology and sensory responses to electrical stimulation
- To familiarize the student with electrode application principles
- To familiarize the student with the application of iontophoresis
- To provide the student with an opportunity to adjust parameters to record the perceived sensation

Equipment

electrical stimulation devices (portable and clinical models)

adjustable parameters (frequency, intensity, ON/OFF times, and so forth)

one pair of large electrodes

    one pair of small electrodes

conductive interface samples for each of the pairs of electrodes (self-adhering, sponges, gel, and so forth)

straps to secure electrodes

iontophoresis unit (electrodes, lead wires, and accessories)

Precautions

in the presence of a fracture

with decreased sensation

in the patient with decreased cognitive ability

during pregnancy

with allergy or skin sensitivity to conductive interface under the electrodes

Contraindications

over the low back or uterus during the first trimester of pregnancy

over a metastases

with osteomyelitis

with thrombosis

in patients who are taking diuretics (these systemically influence ionic balance and regulation)

in patients allergic to iontophoretically delivered medication

LABORATORY EXERCISES

Terminology and Electrodes for Electrical Stimulation

1. Select an electrical stimulator, and identify the following:
   a. Name of the stimulator:

b. Name of the manufacturer:

c. Number of lead wires:

d. Number of available channels:

2. Identify the controls on your stimulator, and indicate the other names that are used to identify them. (You may or may not see all of the following controls on the unit that you select.)
    a. Current type or waveform:

    b. Frequency:

    c. Intensity:

    d. ON/OFF times:

    e. Reciprocal or simultaneous settings:

    f. Pulse duration:

3. Inspect the electrodes that you will be using.
    a. Are they cracked, shiny, uniformly covered?

    b. How many electrodes attach to the lead wire?

There are several common forms of lead wires and electrodes used in the clinic. For electrical stimulation to take place, at least two electrodes need to be in contact with a conductive interface and the patient. These two electrodes must be from one channel of the stimulator.

4. Determine which of the following types of lead/pin setups you have on the stimulator that you have selected.

    a. _____one, two or more stereo jacks

    b. _____one, two or more single-lead jacks

    c. _____a bifurcated lead (lead that has been split and has two pins)

    d. _____pin leads (small diameter and nonadjustable)

    e. _____banana pins (larger diameter and adjustable)

    f. _____other (describe):

5. Determine which of the electrodes will attach securely on your lead wires. Plug in your electrodes so that no metal is showing from the pin.

    a. What conductive interface will you need to use for the electrodes that you have attached?

Sensations and Responses to Electrical Stimulation

1. Select a classmate/patient to receive electrical stimulation to his or her forearm. The area should be assessed for sensation and any abnormalities, such as scars or excessive hair, that may alter the conductivity of the skin.

    Preparation:

    • Check the power cable for any fraying or loose wires.
    • Plug the stimulator into the wall outlet.
    • Turn all outputs to zero.
    • Turn the power ON.
    • Plug the leads that you will be using into the stimulator.
    • Prepare the electrodes for attachment to the patient (whatever is applicable: wet sponges, spread gel, peel off plastic, and so forth).

- Attach the electrodes to your patient (one over the wrist extensor muscle belly, one on the distal extent of the muscle belly).

2. Set the following parameters:

   10 minutes

   100 Hz (or highest available setting for that unit, 80, 90, 100, and so forth)

   200 μsec pulse duration

   Continuous ON time

   a. Gradually increase the intensity, and record the level at which your patient first feels a sensation.

   b. Ask your patient to describe the sensation, and record the response.

   c. Increase the intensity until the sensation is strong, but tolerable, and record it. How high was it in comparison to the initial setting?

   d. Ask your patient to describe how the sensation has changed, and record the response.

3. Decrease the intensity to zero, disconnect the electrodes from the patient, and turn the power OFF.

4. Repeat this exercise until everyone in your group has had a chance to be both the clinician and the patient.

5. Select another stimulator and familiarize yourself with the controls, leads, and electrodes.

6. Preset the following parameters:

   15 minutes

   1 Hz

   200 μsec pulse duration

   continuous ON time

7. Attach the electrodes to the same sites as described previously.

8. Gradually increase the intensity, and record the level at which your patient first feels a sensation.

   a. Ask your patient to describe the sensation, and record your observations with the response.

   b. Slowly increase the intensity until the sensation is strong, but tolerable, and record the level of intensity.

   c. Ask your patient to describe how the sensation has changed, and record the response.

   d. Gradually increase the frequency, and ask the patient to describe how the sensation is changing.

   e. Increase the frequency to 50 Hz, and record your observations.

9. Decrease the intensity to zero, disconnect the electrodes from the patient, and turn the power OFF.
   a. What is the rationale for the sequence that was just described for powering down an electrical stimulator?

Current Density

1. You have been using two equally sized electrodes. Now set up a lead wire so that one electrode is less than half the size of the other electrode on the channel. Place the smaller electrode over the center of the muscle belly and the other electrode distal on the muscle belly. (You may use the forearm again or another muscle group.) Using the same parameters that were selected for the previous exercise, gradually increase the intensity, and record your patient's responses.

   a. Does he or she feel the stimulation underneath both electrodes?

   b. Is that stimulation equally perceived under both electrodes? If not, which one is perceived as stronger, and why?

2. Reverse the electrode setup that you are using. Move the smaller electrode to the distal extent of the muscle belly. Place the larger electrode over the center of the muscle belly.
   a. Gradually increase the intensity, and record your patient's responses.

   b. Does he or she feel the stimulation underneath both electrodes evenly?

   c. Which one is stronger now? Is there a difference in the response, and if so, how?

   d. Why would there be a difference in the sensation?

Iontophoresis

1. Familiarize yourself with the controls and electrodes of the DC stimulator. Also review the contraindications and precautions for application.
   You will notice fewer controls on these units than on the other stimulators you may have used. One control that you will not find on an iontophoresis unit is frequency.
2. Select a classmate/patient who will be receiving iontophoresis of tap water into his or her wrist. The area should be clean and free of cuts, abrasions, and excessive body hair, and the sensation in the area should be intact for all sensations.
3. Prepare each of the electrodes by moistening each one with tap water. Place the active (smaller) electrode over the "anatomic snuffbox" and the remaining, larger electrode over the distal extent of the extensor muscle belly.
   You will also notice that the electrodes are different in size from each other. For iontophoresis, the treatment electrode is approximately half the size of the other electrode. This ensures that a greater concentration of ion flow occurs in the treatment area. This also causes a greater current density under the treatment electrode.
   The goal of iontophoresis is to deliver a known quantity of charge to the patient. This known quantity of charge delivered via ion flow repels the ionic medication of the same polarity into the patient. The goal for quantity of charge is 40 mA minutes. This is calculated by multiplying the output in milliamperes by the time in minutes. If the quantity of charge is high, then the time will be short (4 mA $\times$ 10 minutes = 40 mA minutes). If the quantity of charge is lower, then the time will be longer (1 mA $\times$ 40 minutes = 40 mA minutes). The charge, or inten-

sity, is determined by your patient's tolerance, and when the patient reports that he or she feels a sensation. A patient may or may not feel a sensation from the stimulator during treatment with iontophoresis. If something is felt, it should not be uncomfortable, and the patient may need to be monitored more closely.

4. Connect the leads to the electrodes. If you are administering a medication through the active electrode, then you have to make sure that you connect the lead with the same polarity as the medication to the active electrode. You should also be double checking with the patient that he or she was not allergic to the medication that you are administering.
   a. Slowly increase the intensity. What is it set at?

   b. Based on your intensity level, how long will the unit be ON in order for it to deliver 40 mA minutes?

   c. Ask your patient to describe what, if anything, is felt during the treatment. Is it uncomfortable in any way? Does the patient feel any "pinprick" sensations underneath the electrodes?

5. Once the treatment has finished, slowly decrease the intensity to zero, disconnect the leads from the electrodes, and remove the electrodes from the skin and dispose of them. Observe the skin under both electrodes.
   a. Does the skin from under the electrodes appear any different from the surrounding skin?

   b. Is there a difference between the skin under the positive electrode and the negative electrode?

6. Iontophoresis may cause skin irritation, which can be reduced by moisturizing the skin after treatment. Rub some lotion into the skin that was underneath the electrodes.

Laboratory Questions

1. What terms were used to describe frequency?

2. Which frequency produced a "buzzing" sensation?

3. Which frequency produced a "thumping" sensation?

4. What were the terms used to describe pulse duration?

5. Why didn't the iontophoresis unit have a frequency control or a pulse duration control?

6. What happened when the sensory level of intensity was increased above initial sensation?

7. Why was there a specific sequence for "powering up" and "powering down" the stimulators?

8. What would happen if an electrode fell off during treatment? What would the patient feel?

Electrical Stimulation Devices
Review and Application

Purpose

Electrical stimulation can be one of the most intimidating treatment modalities used in the clinic. Part of the difficulty lies with the terminology used. Electrical stimulation devices seem to have their own specific language that must be learned before you can understand their possibilities. To make matters worse, until fairly recently, there was no "standard" terminology. Consequently, there are sometimes as many as five terms that indicate the same variable, leading to additional confusion.

This laboratory guides the student through the terminology and helps him or her to translate what the terms mean by applying and experiencing them. Students will be adjusting the parameters and learning how to internalize the sensation associated with the terminology.

Students will be applying electrical stimulation to themselves and adjusting the parameters on themselves. Of course, this would not happen in a clinical environment. The purpose of the self-adjustment of electrical parameters is to both familiarize and connect the adjustment with the sensation that it produces.

Objectives

- To provide students with the opportunity to familiarize themselves with electrical stimulation devices and the available parameters
- To provide an individual guided activity for students to discover electrical stimulation for themselves by applying it to themselves and adjusting it for themselves
- To help teach students the language of electrical stimulation

- To help students learn to associate the parameters with the sensation
- To lay the foundation for problem solving with electrical stimulation

Equipment

clinical and portable electrical stimulation units with adjustable parameters:
   pulse duration, frequency, intensity, ramps
electrodes and lead wires appropriate for the electrical stimulation units

Precautions

in areas of decreased sensation
in the patient with decreased
   cognitive ability

during pregnancy
in the presence of a demand-type
   pacemaker

Contraindications

over the low back or uterus during
   the first trimester of pregnancy
over a metastasis
over osteomyelitis

in the area of a thrombus
with patients who are taking
   medications that systemically
   influence ionic balance and
   regulation (diuretics)

LABORATORY EXERCISES

Terminology

1. Select two electrical stimulators. Inspect the units for frayed wiring, biomedical
   engineering stickers of evaluation, and so forth.
   a. Who is the manufacturer of each unit?

   b. What parameters can be adjusted on each unit?

   c. Are there any "preset" parameters?

   d. Are they clinical or portable?

   e. What is the maximum intensity for the units?

2. Record the names of the parameters that the two units use that refer to the same variable (for example, amplitude and intensity, which both refer to the strength of the stimulus).

3. Set one of the units so that:
   The timer is on 10 minutes.
   The intensity is at zero.
   The power is turned ON.
4. Apply one electrode to the web space on the back of one of your hands. The other electrode from the same lead should be applied to the dorsal forearm, over muscle on the same arm.
   a. With all parameters starting at zero (or as low as possible), start increasing the frequency to tolerance (strong, comfortable sensation). What if anything did you feel?

   b. Return the frequency to the starting position.
   c. Now increase the pulse duration from the lowest setting to tolerance. What if anything did you feel?

   d. Return the pulse duration to the starting position.
   e. Increase the intensity from the lowest setting to tolerance. What if anything did you feel?

   f. Return the intensity setting to zero.
5. Preset the pulse duration to 100 μsec. Repeat steps a to f.
6. Preset the frequency to 100 pps. Repeat steps a to f.
   a. Which of the parameters produced a change in sensation when they were increased independently of one another?

   b. Which of the parameters would most accurately tell you "how much" current you were receiving?

7. Set the intensity to a comfortable tingling sensation.
8. Gradually increase the frequency of the unit, and record the sensations that you feel change. Return the frequency to its lowest setting.

9. Gradually increase the pulse duration of the unit, and record the sensations that you feel change. Return the pulse duration to its lowest setting.

10. Gradually increase the intensity above the comfortable tingling sensation. What happens to the sensation?

11. Set the unit so that:
    The pulse duration is 100 μsec.
    The frequency is 50 pps.
    The intensity is at the zero starting point.
    a. Collect the following data:
       • When you increase the intensity, at what amount do you first feel something?

       • Is that sensation tingling, a contraction, or a sharp pain?

12. Set the unit so that:
    The pulse duration is 200 μsec.
    The frequency is 50 pps.
    The intensity is at the zero starting point.
    a. Collect the following data:
       - When you increase the intensity, at what amount do you first feel something?

       - Is that sensation tingling, a contraction, or a sharp pain?

13. Set the unit so that:
    The pulse duration is at the zero starting point.
    The frequency is 50 pps.
    The intensity is as high as possible.
    a. Collect the following data:
       - When you increase the pulse duration, at what duration do you first feel something?

       - Is that sensation tingling, a contraction, or a sharp pain?

14. Fill in the chart in Figure 5–1 with the data that you have collected. (Intensity is on the vertical axis, and pulse duration is on the horizontal axis.)

Strength Duration Curve Findings

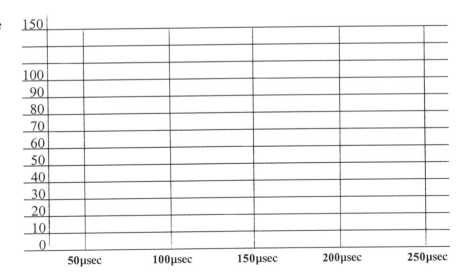

Pulse Duration in microseconds (μsec)

Figure 5–1

- Use dots for tingling sensation.
- Use triangles for contraction.
- Use squares for sharp pain.

15. Set the unit so that:
    The pulse duration is 200 μsec.
    The frequency is 50 pps.
    The intensity is at the zero starting point.

16. Place one electrode on the back of the web space of your hand, and place the other electrode from the same channel on the dorsal forearm.

17. Gradually increase the intensity until there is a motor response.

18. Leaving the intensity at this level, gradually decrease the frequency to 1 pps.
    a. How did the sensation change?

    b. What is occurring now that didn't occur with the frequency at 50 pps?

19. Gradually increase the intensity.
    a. What happens to the response?

    b. Describe the sensation in terminology that a patient would understand.

20. Gradually increase the frequency. What happens?

21. Increase the frequency to 50 pps, and stay there for 1 minute.
22. Increase the frequency to 100 pps, and stay there for about 5 minutes.
    a. Describe the sensation.

    b. What happens to the motor response?

Laboratory Questions

1. If you were treating a patient with electrical stimulation and you were using a portable unit that had adjustable parameters, what would you do if the intensity were turned up as high as possible and the patient still did not feel the stimulus?

2. The chart that you filled in was actually a strength duration curve. Answer the following questions based on the information in the chart:
    • Which of the sensations required the least amount of intensity to elicit?

    • Which of the sensations required the shortest pulse duration to elicit?

    • What would it mean if a patient started to have a twitching-type contraction?

    • What would the minimum pulse duration be, how high would the intensity be, and what would the frequency be to produce the twitching type of contraction?

3. When turning off an electrical stimulator, which controls should be returned to zero. Why?

4. When turning off an electrical stimulator, which controls may be left alone?

5. If you were adjusting the intensity and the patient reported that he or she felt the current very strongly just after you started to increase it, what would be the possible explanations for this?

6. You are increasing the intensity on a unit, and after increasing it to the maximum level, the patient still reports feeling little or no sensation. What would be the possible cause and remedies?

7. You are setting up an electrical stimulation unit, and while adjusting the unit, the patient reports feeling a throbbing sensation under the electrodes. What would be the possible cause and remedies?

8. If you had to explain the parameter terminology to a patient, what would you say that each of the controls represents in terms of the sensations that the patient will feel?

9. If a patient reports to you feeling sharp knifelike sensation underneath the electrodes, what would be the possible causes and remedies?

Electrical Stimulation for Pain Relief
Sensory Analgesia

Purpose

This laboratory exercise has been designed to familiarize the student with the application and expected patient responses to transcutaneous electrical nerve stimulation (TENS) for the relief of pain. It will also familiarize the student with electrode placement site selection and stimulation parameters for sensory analgesia. Students will have the opportunity to experience varied parameters on both portable and clinical stimulation devices.

Objectives

- To familiarize students with electrode placement site selection guidelines
- To provide the student with the opportunity to experience TENS as both a patient and a clinician
- To build on the students understanding of the setting and selection of stimulation parameters
- To provide the student with the opportunity to experience both self-adjustment of intensity with electrical stimulation and clinician adjustment of the intensity

Equipment

TENS stimulators (clinical and portable models)
lead wires for the stimulators
electrically conductive gel or self-adhering electrodes

four equally sized electrodes
cloth or paper tape to secure electrodes
electrical stimulators capable of producing pulse durations in excess of 1 msec

Precautions

during pregnancy

in patients with known cardiac disease

in the presence of malignancy

directly over an open wound

in patients with impaired cognition

in patients with peripheral neuropathies

Contraindications

during the first trimester of pregnancy

over a metastasis, unless the condition has been diagnosed as terminal

in patients with demand-type pacemaker

over the carotid sinus

over the eye

in patients with epilepsy

in patients with undiagnosed pain syndromes

for transcranial application

LABORATORY EXERCISES

Transcutaneous Electrical Nerve Stimulation Electrode Placements and Their Sensations

1. Familiarize yourself with the TENS unit that you have selected by reviewing both the controls on the stimulator and the instruction manual for the device.
   a. What are the available ranges of parameters?
      - Frequency:

      - Pulse duration:

      - Intensity:

   b. Are there any other controls on the device? If yes, what are they, and what do they do?

2. Familiarize yourself with electrode placement site charts in the department and in your textbooks or recommended readings.
   a. What are the types or names of the points that exhibit decreased resistance to the flow of electrical current?

b. What are some of your options for electrode placement sites if your patient had been referred to the department for lower back pain?

c. Record the location of four paraspinal electrode placement sites around L4–5.

3. Prepare the electrodes and the unit to be applied to your patient. Select a classmate/patient for TENS application to the lower back. Position your patient so that the low back is exposed and accessible to you.

    Apply one channel of electrodes to the right side and one channel to the left side of the paraspinal musculature, using the sites that you identified from the charts. Preset the parameters for sensory analgesia. (Consult your book and lecture notes.) Slowly increase the intensity of the first channel, and ask your patient to let you know when they first feel a sensation, where they feel it, how it feels, and when the intensity is strong, but tolerable.

    Gradually increase the intensity of the second channel, and repeat the same sequence. Assess the area vertically in between the electrodes.

    a. Were the intensity levels equal on both sides? What would explain this?

    b. Does your patient feel any sensation in between the electrodes? What would explain this?

4. Turn both intensities OFF, leave the electrodes in place, and disconnect the pin tips from the leads. This time, connect the leads to the electrodes so that there is one channel above L4–5 and one channel below. Repeat the same steps.

5. Turn both intensities OFF, leave the electrodes in place, and disconnect the pin tips from the leads. This time, connect the leads to the electrodes so that there is one channel crisscrossing the other channel. Repeat the same steps.

    a. Did any of the setups produce more sensory stimulation than the others? Why or why not?

b. When would the selection of acupuncture points for electrode placement sites be considered appropriate?

c. What other options are available for electrode placement site selection? (Describe at least two and give the rationale for each.)

Intensity Adjustment and Patient Instructions for Sensory Analgesia

1. Select a classmate/patient to have TENS applied to the shoulder. Select electrode placement sites that would encompass the entire shoulder, and provide sensory analgesia throughout the local area.
   a. Describe your electrode placement.

   b. What is your rationale for your selections?

2. Preset the parameters on the unit for sensory analgesia. Instruct your patient how and what to adjust to increase the intensity of the stimulation. Also, instruct the

patient in how and where to apply the electrodes, replace the battery, care for the TENS unit and electrodes, self-assess their level of discomfort, and record the assessment results.

Give the patient the TENS unit and ask him or her to increase the intensity to a strong, but comfortable, level. The patient should increase the intensity if the sensation "fades" at all after the initial setup.

a. How did the setting of the intensity differ when the patient adjusted it?

b. What would be a possible rationale for instructing a patient how to adjust and care for a TENS unit?

c. What additional considerations would there be for unit selection for a patient so that the patient could adjust the intensity?

d. Would you expect the intensity for sensory analgesia to change while it was on? Why or why not?

e. What would happen if you increased the pulse duration of the stimulation?

f. Would this ever be indicated? Why or why not?

3. Instruct your patient how to terminate treatment, reassess the treatment area, and remove the electrodes.

Low-Rate Stimulation for Analgesia

1. Select a classmate/patient for application of motor-level stimulation to the triceps surae bilaterally. Position your patient so that he or she is comfortable and supported, with the ankle free to plantarflex and dorsiflex. Consult charts either in your books or in the department for electrode placement sites, and apply the electrodes to elicit a motor response from the triceps surae. Preset your TENS unit for motor-level stimulation at a low rate. Gradually increase the intensity until a twitch response is visible. Now increase the intensity to the highest tolerable level so that joint movement is visible.

   a. What are the differences between this level of stimulation and sensory analgesia?

   b. How long would it take for a patient to report some decrease in pain following this mode of stimulation?

   c. What are your patient's subjective responses to this mode of stimulation?

   d. When might this mode be considered appropriate for a patient?

   e. What is the mechanism for pain relief that this mode is intended to induce?

f. Do you expect the patient to adapt to this mode of stimulation? Why or why not?

g. How long is the carryover time for relief expected from this mode of stimulation?

h. What possible rationale would there be for distally placed electrodes if this setup were recommended for lower back pain?

Hyperstimulation Analgesia or Noxious-Level Stimulation

1. Familiarize yourself with the stimulator. It must be capable of producing pulse durations greater than 1 msec. Select a classmate/patient for electroacupuncture to the web space on the back of the hand. Position your patient comfortably, and position yourself so that you are at eye level with the patient.

    There is probably a resistance meter of some form on the stimulator. It may measure conductance or resistance. Familiarize yourself with it by touching the two ends of the leads together and noting what the meter reads. Then hold the larger electrode in your hand, and touch yourself with the probe electrode. Compare the meter reading to your first reading. If it was lower, then the meter was reading conductance. If the second meter reading was higher, then it was reading resistance. Preset the parameters on the stimulator to 4 Hz, at least 1 msec pulse duration and 30 seconds of ON time.

    Give the patient the dispersive/inactive electrode to hold in his or her other hand. You will not need gel or a conductive interface because the patient will be grasping the electrode in the palm of the hand, which usually perspires when grasping something rubber. The perspiration will serve as the contact medium. Patients also tend to perspire when they are told that what they are going to experience will be a sensation similar to a "hot needle" or bee sting.

    Locate the area that is most electrically active within the web space on the back of your patient's hand. This would be the most conductive area (HoKu or LI 4). Once it has been identified, press the ON button, and gradually increase the intensity while watching your patient's eyes. The amount of dilation of the pupils will change when the stimulus is as strong as the patient can tolerate it. Restart the timer for 30 seconds. It is intended to be noxious. After the 30 seconds is up, remove the probe, and ask your patient to describe what was felt. Repeat for all members of your group.

a. When would this mode of stimulation be indicated?

b. What would you need to explain to the patient to ensure that your chances of having it work would be enhanced?

c. What possible explanations would there be for positioning yourself at eye level with your patient?

d. Why would this type of stimulator have a conductance/resistance meter?

e. How did the sensation of the stimulus differ from sensory analgesia?

PATIENT SCENARIOS

Read through the patient scenarios, and determine the following:
- Whether or not electrical stimulation would be indicated for pain relief
- What precautions there might be for the patient described
- What the parameters would be for the patient and your rationale for those parameters

- Where the electrodes should be placed, how many of them should be placed, and why
- Whether more than one mode would be indicated for pain relief
- Whether or not the patient may benefit from home use of a portable stimulator (and your rationale)

Case Study A

Mr. George has been referred to the physical therapy department for pain relief. He has been diagnosed with herpes zoster, and on examination, there is a large inflamed area on his left side. It starts midline posteriorly in the thoracic region and extends anteriorly, tracing the last five ribs to the sternum. He is 85 years old, lives alone, and is otherwise healthy, aside from an ulcer that has been controlled successfully by diet and medication for over 20 years. His primary complaints are hypersensitivity to light touch throughout the inflamed area. It is so sensitive that he now guards the area by flexing his trunk so that his clothing does not touch his skin on the left side.

Case Study B

James is a maintenance engineer for a retirement community. He has been referred to the physical therapy department for pain relief subsequent to a low-back injury he suffered while at work. He is a 42-year-old "workaholic" who has been performing strengthening exercises to stabilize his back. He has also worked through a "work hardening program," and he is exceedingly anxious to return to work. His only limitation is chronic low-back pain. He is an avid bicyclist, canoeist, and hiker. He is looking for relief that would not interfere with his work with lawnmowers, power tools, and mechanical equipment.

Case Study C

Carol is a cartoonist who has been referred to the physical therapy department for pain management techniques subsequent to a cervical strain injury. She was involved in a motor vehicle accident in which she was hit from behind. She now has muscle guarding and marked decreases in her cervical range of motion in all directions. Her primary complaint is occipital headaches. She lives alone and works from a home office. Most of her day is spent at an artist's table that is angled at 45°. Medications to reduce muscle guarding and inflammation caused other complications in conjunction with medications that she was taking for depression.

DOCUMENTATION

Electrical stimulation can be used to control and reduce discomfort. Because electrical stimulation can be used in a variety of ways to accomplish these goals, it is important to document what produced favorable results for a patient. Documentation should include the following information:

Treatment goal:	sensory analgesia or pain management
Pre-treatment pain assessment:	visual analog or other quantifiable measure
Post-treatment pain assessment:	same instrument that was applied pre-treatment
Electrode placement sites:	only if there was some "trial and error" before sites proved themselves to be successful
Stimulation parameters:	only if there was some "trial and error" before parameters proved themselves to be successful
Specific stimulator used:	only if there was some "trial and error" surrounding the device that was selected (Include the manufacturer if home use of the device was recommended.)

Select two of the "patients" that you applied modalities to during the laboratory exercise, and write a progress note that includes the patient's subjective complaints, objective information that you recorded, the physical agent that was applied, the manner of application, the response to the applied physical agent, and your assessment.

Laboratory Questions

1. What was the most comfortable mode of stimulation for your patients?

2. What was the most uncomfortable mode of stimulation?

3. Which of the parameters would have accomplished A beta fiber stimulation?

4. What would the necessary parameters be for C fiber stimulation, and when might this be indicated?

5. Your patient has increased the intensity to the highest level for a portable TENS unit, and he or she still does not feel the stimulation. What are the possible remedies, which would you employ first, and why?

6. Discuss the potential success rate when using TENS as the sole technique to treat a patient.

7. Discuss the similarities and differences between the various electrode placement site selection options and provide the rationale for each of the options.

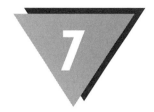

Electrical Stimulation for Motor Responses
Therapeutic Application of Neuromuscular Electrical Stimulation

Purpose

This laboratory exercise has been developed to introduce the student to a variety of electrically induced motor responses. Stimulation parameters and electrode placement sites for motor responses are different than for other treatment goals. This will familiarize students with the sensory differences as well as the importance of accurate descriptions of these sensations when instructing patients what they should and should not feel during the stimulation.

Objectives

- To integrate the understanding of the application of specific treatment parameters with the accomplishment of specific treatment goals
- To integrate the concepts of appropriate electrode placement site selection with goal accomplishment
- To compare electrical stimulation parameters and electrode placement sites for edema reduction, muscle spasm reduction, and muscle strengthening

Equipment

electrical stimulation devices with
   adjustable pulse durations, ON/OFF
   times, frequencies, ON/OFF ramps
lead wires
straps to secure electrodes

electrically conductive electrode
   interface
reusable or self-adhering electrodes
   (optional)

Precautions

pregnancy
malignancies
insensate areas

fractures
patient history of cardiac disease

Contraindications

during the first trimester of pregnancy
over or around a metastasis
across an unstable, nonunion, or acute
   fracture
in the presence of a thrombus

in patients with demand-
   type pacemakers
in patients with active
   tuberculosis
over or around the carotid sinus

LABORATORY EXERCISES

Motor Responses to Electrical Stimulation

EDEMA REDUCTION

1. Select a classmate/patient for electrical stimulation to elicit a motor response in
   his or her calf. Position your patient as if he or she had an acutely sprained edematous ankle. Determine where the electrodes should be placed to elicit muscle
   contractions in both the agonists and antagonists for dorsiflexion. Indicate the
   electrode placement sites that you will be using.

2. Select a stimulator capable of producing levels of stimulation that elicit a tetanic
   muscle contraction. (The device should have longer pulse durations, 1–80 pps frequency range, ON/OFF times, relatively high intensity levels, and reciprocal
   modes of stimulation.) Familiarize yourself with the stimulator and preset parameters, and identify the parameters that you will be using:
   a. Frequency

b. Pulse duration

3. Prepare and apply the electrodes that you have selected. They should be appropriately sized relative to the sizes of the muscles that you will be stimulating. Remember that electrode size influences the ease of eliciting a comfortable muscle contraction. Large electrodes have generally lower resistance levels, which translate into lower intensities necessary to elicit a muscle contraction. (Try eliciting a contraction with small electrodes and then with electrodes twice that size.)

4. Adjust the intensities of each of the channels separately, making sure that you are in the reciprocating mode and increasing the intensity only for the channel that is ON.

   a. How much more intensity was necessary to elicit a muscle contraction than was necessary for the patient to report that a stimulus was felt?

   b. What happens to the quality of the contraction as you slowly increase the frequency up to 80 pps (during the ON times)?

   c. What happens to the quality of the contraction as you slowly decrease the frequency down to 10 pps (during the ON times)?

   d. What was the "optimal frequency" for the muscles that you were stimulating?

   e. Was it the same for both the agonist and the antagonist? Why or why not?

   f. What do you believe is the purpose for reciprocating channels of stimulation? (Try a simultaneous mode of stimulation, and observe what happens.)

g. Why would a reciprocating mode of stimulation to the agonist and antagonist muscle groups that cross an edematous area be used in assisting edema reduction? What would the potential rationale be?

REDUCTION OF MUSCLE GUARDING

1. Whenever an injury occurs to soft tissue, one of the natural responses that takes place is muscle guarding, which acts to protect the area from further movement or injury. Muscle guarding impedes the circulation to the area and promotes metabolite retention. This may increase pain perception owing to the sensitization of the nociceptors by the presence of metabolic by-products. Reduction in muscle guarding may cause a reduction in pain.
2. Select a classmate/patient for electrical stimulation to the upper trapezius muscles bilaterally. Position your patient so that he or she is comfortable and the upper trapezei are in a resting position. (If your patient has some palpable muscle tightness, assess the degree of tightness and tenderness to palpation.)
3. Identify the parameters that you will need to elicit a tetanic muscle contraction, and select the electrodes that you will be using. Apply the electrodes in each of the following setup configurations:

(1)		(2)		(3)	
O	X	X	X	X	O
X	O	O	O	X	O

a. First try each of the setups with reciprocal ON/OFF times and 3-second ON ramps. Which was the most comfortable for your patient?

b. Then choose a simultaneous ON time for each of the setups. Was there a difference in the sensation for any of the three setups? Why or why not?

c. Which is more comfortable, using ON ramps or not using them? Why?

d. If your goal was to decrease muscle guarding specifically in the upper trapezius muscles bilaterally, which setup would be most logical for accomplishing your goal?

e. If your goal was to decrease the muscle's ability to maintain a contraction, what parameters would you adjust and what would be your rationale for adjusting them?

f. If your patient for this exercise had palpable muscle tightness before you applied the stimulation, reassess the tightness. Was there a noticeable change to you, to the patient?

MUSCLE STRENGTHENING

1. Electrical stimulation has been used successfully for the enhancement of an isometric muscle contraction. It is one of the tools used in a comprehensive treatment plan for postoperative recovery for several orthopedic procedures. The key components of this form of stimulation include the isolation of the muscle group and the stabilization of the joint that the muscle acts on.
2. Select a classmate/patient for electrical stimulation to the vastus medialis and the rectus femoris. Position your patient so that he or she is supported in about 20° of knee flexion and no joint motion is permitted. (You may use a commercial dynamometer to stabilize the joint isometrically or devise some other means to stabilize the joint.)
3. Set up the stimulator that you have selected so that you will be able to elicit strong muscle contractions. Identify electrode placement sites for both muscles, and apply the electrodes securely, one channel for each muscle.
4. Slowly increase the intensity of the stimulus until a strong muscle contraction is elicited.
   a. What should the patient feel? Does the patient feel it?

b. What would make the stimulus more comfortable for your patient?

5. Try one of your potential solutions for comfort. Does it make a difference?

a. How much intensity can your patient tolerate?

b. What is the optimal frequency for a tetanic contraction for this patient?

c. What would the rationale be for a 10-second ON time and 50-second OFF time?

d. Does the quality of the muscle contraction that you are eliciting change with successive contractions? If yes, how?

e. What happens to the sensation of the stimulation if the patient contracts with the stimulation?

6. Try other options that you believe may make the stimulus more tolerable for your patient. Observe the responses. What was the "best" setup or option for your patient?

FUNCTIONAL ELECTRICAL STIMULATION

Electrical stimulation has been used to augment muscle function in a wide variety of areas, including urinary incontinence, shoulder subluxations, footdrop during gate, and standing stability for the paraplegic patient population. One of the common elements to these applications is the development of portable "intelligent" technology that is capable of producing the necessary parameters when the patient needs them and in a way that does not actually interfere with a patient's ability to perform the activity itself. For example, the technology has been in existence for years to elicit a muscle contraction with electrical stimulation; however, a 6-foot power cord was usually necessary to provide the power source of stimulation. Devices are now much more portable and accessible for patients than they ever have been.

1. Select a classmate/patient for electrical stimulation to their middle deltoid and supraspinatus. You will be adjusting the parameters so that you can elicit a tetanic muscle contraction to help reduce a subluxation of the humoral head. Position your patient so that he or she will be able to see what you are doing. Teach the patient the electrode placement sites that he or she will need to use and how to assess success in eliciting the desired response.

2. Familiarize yourself and the patient with the portable stimulator that you will be using. Teach your patient how to inspect the treatment area and the unit, care for and apply the electrodes, and adjust the intensity controls. Determine the appropriate ON/OFF timing for your patient and whether or not ON ramps are functional for this patient. Turn the unit ON, and have the patient set the intensity level.

   a. Why do you think that you were instructed to teach the patient so much during this lab activity?

   b. How much more time did it take to do the "teaching"?

   c. What parameters did you use (that is, frequency, pulse duration, ON/OFF times, ramps)?

   d. Which is more important, a specific intensity reading or a specific response? Why?

PATIENT SCENARIOS

Read through the patient scenarios, and determine the following:
- Whether electrical stimulation would be indicated or not and your rationale for your response
- What the parameters for stimulation should be for the patient if electrical stimulation is indicated
- Where the electrode placement sites should be
- What additional considerations that there might be for a patient to be considered a good candidate for electrical stimulation
- Whether the electrical stimulation should be applied clinically or at home and why

Case Study A

Mary is a 55-year-old woman who has been admitted to the rehabilitation hospital subsequent to an unsuccessful attempt to reduce the effects of arteriosclerosis in her carotid arteries. She has had bilateral cerebrovascular accidents (CVAs) as a result of the procedures performed. She is otherwise healthy, with no previous medical complications. She has been referred for physical therapy to see whether electrical stimulation can be used to reduce the subluxation of her right shoulder. She is alternatively expressively and receptively aphasic and has limited manual dexterity skills. Presently, she is nonambulatory because of balance difficulties and an inability to use her upper extremities for support with assistive devices.

Case Study B

Joe is a 48-year-old shoemaker who has been referred to the physical therapy department subsequent to a CVA. He presently has flexor spasticity in his right upper extremity, and he has footdrop on the right. His goal is ambulation without the short leg brace that he has been ambulating with for the last 3 months since the CVA.

Case Study C

Cynthia is a legal secretary who has been referred to the physical therapy department subsequent to injuries that she sustained in an automobile accident 3 days ago. She has a cervical strain with pronounced muscle guarding throughout the cervical spine, shown by limitations in active range of motion in all directions. She also is scheduled to have a medial meniscectomy next week. Her physician and employer are concerned about her ability to return to work after the knee surgery and want her to be as prepared as she can be preoperatively to ensure a prompt return to work. (She is an aerobics instructor at night and a long-distance bicycle racer, with a race in 2 months.)

Case Study D

Mike is an athletic trainer for the track team of a local high school. He has been referred to physical therapy for edema reduction for his left ankle, which has now been sprained for total of six times in the last 3 years. His attempts at icing the joint have not been successful in reducing the edema. He has lateral instability and marked weakness in the ankle invertors and evertors on the left. Mike is well motivated and has no other medical complications.

DOCUMENTATION

Documentation of treatments rendered with electrical stimulation involves the recording of the treatment goal for which the stimulation was applied and the result. Documentation of electrode placement sites, parameters, or stimulator used would be necessary only if there were some significant trial-and-error period before optimal results were achieved and if there were some unusual techniques used to accomplish the results. For example, if a patient had tendon transplant surgery, it would be important to know where the electrode placement sites were located.

Once the goal is identified, the parameters to accomplish the goal and the electrode placement sites necessary should be fairly obvious to other clinicians who may be reading the documentation to duplicate the treatment rendered.

Select two of the "patients" that you applied modalities to during the laboratory exercise, and write a progress note that includes each patient's subjective complaints, the objective information that you recorded, the physical agent that was applied and manner of application, the response to the applied physical agent, and your assessment.

Laboratory Questions

1. What was the optimal frequency to accomplish a tetanic contraction?

 • How did your optimal frequency compare with those of your classmates?

 • Of what significance is an optimal frequency?

 • What were some of the common factors for the applications of electrical stimulation performed during this laboratory exercise?

2. If you had two stimulators to choose from, and one had a maximum pulse duration of 100 μsec and the other stimulator had a maximum pulse duration of 200 μsec,

which one would require a lower intensity to elicit a tetanic muscle contraction? Why?

3. Of what potential value are ON ramps?

4. Why is it more difficult to adjust parameters other than the intensity on portable functional electrical stimulators?

5. What do you think would be the most significant barriers to the successful use of functional electrical stimulation for gait? How would you potentially overcome them?

6. What objective measures could you employ to ensure that the level of electrical stimulation consistently elicited the same level of muscle contraction response?

7. Describe the necessary parameters for electrical stimulation to maintain muscle strength.

Therapeutic Application of Interferential Current Therapy

Purpose

This laboratory exercise is designed to familiarize the student with the proper application techniques of different forms of interferential current (IFC) therapy. It will build on skills attained in prior laboratory exercises and help to solidify the use of electrotherapy devices. It is also intended to strengthen the processes necessary to achieve optimal therapeutic results with electrical stimulation devices.

Objectives

- To familiarize the student with the application of IFC electrical stimulation devices
- To provide students with the opportunity to feel and apply interferential electrical stimulation
- To provide the student with opportunities to determine electrode placement sites and parameter selection to accomplish a therapeutic treatment goal and test out the selections

Equipment

IFC generator
six electrodes (four of equal size)
sponges, gel, and straps to secure electrodes or self-adhering/reusable electrodes

Precautions

pregnancy
malignancy
insensate areas
fractures

Contraindications

during the first trimester of pregnancy

over or around a malignancy

across an unstable or nonunion fracture

in the presence of a thrombus

for transcranial application of
electrodes

for transthoracic application of
electrodes across the heart

LABORATORY EXERCISES

Interferential Current Electrode Placement Sites and Target Treatment Areas

Interferential current requires the use of two separate generators that produce a frequency greater than 1000 Hz. The devices produce 2000, 4000, or 5000 Hz, which is referred to as the *carrier frequency* of the stimulator. Familiarize yourselves with the device you will be using, and determine what parameters are available and how you would adjust them.

- What is the carrier frequency of the device you are using?

- Are other carrier frequencies available on the device you are using, and if so what are they?

- What would be the appropriate pulse burst rate, or *beat frequency,* for sensory analgesia? For a tetanic motor response?

There are two forms of IFC: frequency difference and full field. Both forms can be used to provide sensory and generalized dynamic motor responses throughout a treatment area. Frequency-difference IFC uses two generators that produce carrier frequencies that vary slightly from one another. If one channel is producing 4000 Hz and the other channel, which is set up to intersect with it, is producing 4035 Hz, then the tissue responds as it would to 35 Hz. It is more accurately referred to as a beat frequency of 35. The area underneath the electrodes experiences a decrease in sensation, referred to as *Wedensky inhibition* (named after the individual who initially described the phenomenon). There is an asynchronous firing of the sensory nerve fibers, resulting in a loss of sensation or numbness. The actual treatment area where the current is perceived lies deep within the tissues, where the current pathways intersect each other.

- What would the beat frequency be if the difference between the two carriers were 120 Hz?

1. Select a classmate/patient for electrical stimulation to the knee. You will be applying IFC for generalized pain reduction throughout the knee joint, as if your patient had been diagnosed with chondromalacia of the patella that was producing pain posterior to the patella and inflammation on the superior medial aspect of the knee joint.
2. Position your patient so that the knee is supported in about 20° of flexion. Set up the electrodes (four electrodes of equal size) so that they crisscross over the knee on both the medial and the lateral aspects of the knee.
3. Slowly increase the intensity controls on both channels, and ask your patient to describe *what* he or she is feeling and *where* he or she is feeling it.

    a. What happens to the sensation when your patient increases knee flexion to about 90°?

    b. Does the patient still feel it in the same area?

    c. Can the patient tolerate more intensity now? (If yes, increase the intensity.)

4. Locate the control on the device that will make the current have a dynamic component. Turn it on, and ask your patient to describe what he or she is feeling now.

    a. Is it easier or more difficult for your patient to locate the stimulus than it was before you added the dynamic component to the IFC?

b. Can the patient tolerate more intensity now? (If yes, increase the intensity.)

5. Record the intensity level, and turn the intensity down on both of the channels. Reverse the position of one of the channels of electrodes. Use the same sites, but switch the two electrodes. Gradually increase the intensity until the patient reports the same sensation that was felt before. If possible, bring the intensity up to the same level that it was at before.
a. Does it feel the same as it did before?

b. Would you expect there to be a difference in the sensation? Why or why not?

"Nerve Block" Sensory Analgesia

1. Select a classmate/patient for electrical stimulation to the elbow. You will be performing a transverse friction massage to the common extensor tendon on the lateral epicondyle. Assess the amount of discomfort that the patient feels when you deeply palpate the lateral epicondyle and rub transverse to the tendon. You will be using electrical stimulation to assist in blocking the pain produced by the transverse friction massage.

   Interferential current uses a carrier frequency in the range of several thousand hertz. A numbness results from an asynchronous firing of the sensory nerve fibers. The effects of IFC actually result from the crossing of two separate current generator pathways within the tissue. There is no sensation directly underneath the electrodes except for a paresthesia, which lasts only as long as the stimulus is applied.

   If the two separate generators from an IFC unit were *not* crossed, there would be no "interference" of the generators. It is feasible that one could create the numbness in a specific area with precise electrode placement. Current follows the path of least resistance, which is often parallel to anatomic structures.
2. Place one channel from the generator so that the electrodes are superior and inferior to the common extensor origin on the lateral epicondyle. Place the other channel so that the electrodes are on the flexor surface of the forearm.
3. Slowly increase the intensity on both of the channels until it is strong, but tolerable, to your patient. Wait about 2 minutes, and then see if you can increase the intensity.
4. Repalpate the common extensor tendon, and compare the sensation to the initial palpation response.
a. Was your patient "as sensitive" once the stimulator was on for a few minutes?

b. Does the intensity of the stimulator seem to "fade out" frequently? Why would you or why wouldn't you expect this to occur?

5. Turn the intensity level down, and crisscross the electrodes from the two channels. Set a pulse burst rate, or beat frequency, of 2 Hz. Return the intensity level to what it was set at before, and ask your patient to describe what he or she is feeling now.

    a. Is the sensation that the patient is feeling now more like a "buzzing" or "thumping" sensation?

    b. What would you say to prepare the patient for the sensation?

6. Repalpate the lateral epicondyle, and compare the sensation to the initial palpation response.
    a. Has the sensation changed at all since the first time that your palpated it?

    b. Would you expect it to have changed? Why or why not?

Motor-Level Responses with Interferential Current

1. Select a classmate/patient to have electrical stimulation to the shoulder. You will be setting up the electrodes as if your patient had an adhesive capsulitis of the shoulder. Place one channel of electrodes from the anterior axillary fold to the posterior axillary fold. Place the other channel of electrodes so that one electrode is on the insertion of the deltoid and the other electrode is on the middle of the superior border of the upper trapezius.
    a. What would the target tissue area be with this electrode placement setup?

    b. If the IFC unit were capable of eliciting a motor response, what muscles do you think would respond?

2. Select a pulse burst rate, or beat frequency, that would be capable of eliciting a tetanic muscle contraction. Slowly increase the intensity levels in both sets of electrodes until the stimulus is strong, but tolerable, for the patient.
   a. Is there a palpable motor response occurring?

   b. Can your patient tolerate more intensity after a few minutes? (If yes, increase it.)

3. Adjust the IFC to add the dynamic component of the current.
   a. Describe what, if anything, happens.

4. Increase the intensity to see if you can elicit more of a response.
   a. What does the response "look like" to you?

   b. Which muscles are responding, if any?

5. Decrease the intensity to zero, and reverse one of the channels of electrodes. Increase the intensity to where it was before.
   a. Will there be any difference since you switched one of the channels of electrodes? Why or why not?

   b. Does your patient describe the sensation as being any different?

   c. If different muscles did respond, what could have caused that to occur?

    d. If different muscles didn't respond, what could have caused that to occur?

6. Ask your patient to try to reposition the shoulder, and note how the sensation changes if at all.
    a. 90° of shoulder flexion

    b. 90° of internal rotation

    c. 90° of external rotation

    d. Hyperextension

    e. End range of flexion

    f. Horizontal adduction and abduction

Electrode Size and Current Concentration

1. Select a classmate/patient for IFC electrical stimulation to the upper cervical spine. You will be setting up your patient as if the patient had been referred to the

physical therapy department for injuries sustained in an automobile accident. Your patient complains of occipital headaches and has restricted cervical range of motion in all directions because of pain and muscle guarding.

2. Position your patient so that the cervical spine is in a neutral position and at rest. Try the following:

   a. Apply IFC to the cervical spine with one electrode from each of the channels placed suboccipitally, just below the hairline. Place the other electrode from each of the channels over the insertion of the levator scapula. Use four electrodes of equal size, and cross the channels to produce the interference of the current pathways within the tissue. Increase the intensity, and ask your patient to describe what he or she feels and where he or she is feeling it.

   b. Apply IFC to the same sites as in a, but place smaller electrodes suboccipitally. Is there a difference? Why or why not? What effect does the size of the electrode have on the current density?

   c. Apply IFC to the same sites as in a, but place the smaller electrodes over the levator scapulae insertions and the larger electrodes suboccipitally. Is there a difference? Why or why not?

PATIENT SCENARIOS

Read through the patient scenarios, and determine the following:
- Whether IFC would be indicated, and if yes, what your treatment goal would be for the device
- What application techniques you would use for the patient (position, electrode types, sizes, and placement sites)
- What precautions there would be for the patient described
- What additional information, if any, you would need to know prior to treating the patient
- How you would assess whether the technique you selected is appropriate

Case Study A

Bill is an avid cyclist who was recently involved in an automobile accident while riding his bike. He sustained a midshaft femoral fracture, numerous contusions, abrasions, and a cervical and lumbar strain. His lower left extremity is casted, and he is ambulating NWB on the L leg with crutches. His primary complaints are of severe headaches and an inability to hold his head up while typing or trying to work at his desk. He is a college professor.

Case Study B

Marcy is an executive secretary who was referred to the physical therapy department for recurring bilateral lateral epicondylitis. She has been treated previously with injections of cortisone and has had no significant reduction in her discomfort. She complains of a "gripping" sensation with active wrist extension. Marcy has a family history of diabetes, and both of her parents have been diagnosed with different forms of cancer within the past year.

Case Study C

Al is an occupational therapist who recently had a below-the-knee lower extremity amputation. His stump is hypersensitive and edematous, making it difficult for him to be fitted for a prosthesis. The amputation is a result of a traumatic crushing injury to the lower leg. He has no significant medical history that would complicate his recovery except his lack of patience.

Case Study D

Roger is an advertising executive who recently underwent open heart surgery in which he had a total of four bypasses performed. He is complaining of sternal pain and inflammation. It is now 1 month after his surgery, and he is considered to be medically stable. Prior to the surgery, he led a sedentary lifestyle.

Case Study E

Kevin, a father of two active boys, has a recurring traumatic chondromalacia of the patella. He initially injured both knees by falling directly onto the patellae while playing touch football. There is significant inflammation surrounding both the superior medial and the lateral aspects of both knees. There is palpable crepitous with active knee extension. His primary complaints include pain, decreased strength, and an inability to "trust" his knees. He has no significant other medical history.

Case Study F

Joan has been diagnosed as having piriformis syndrome. Evidently her sciatic radiating pain is caused by a chronic spasm of the hip rotators. She has been referred to the physical therapy department to see what can be done to help relieve her radiating pain. Joan is employed as a package delivery person and truck driver and is anxious to return to work.

DOCUMENTATION

Interferential current is a form of electrical stimulation that can be used to treat a variety of clinical symptoms. The treatment goal is more important for documentation purposes than the form of electrical stimulation used.

Documentation should include the following:

- Treatment goal for the device
- Area being treated
- Treatment time
- Any objective measures that were initially used to determine the modality of choice
- Results of the treatment intervention
- Electrode placement sites should be documented *only* if significant trial and error of electrode placement took place before result could be achieved

Select two of the "patients" that you applied modalities to during the laboratory exercise, and write a progress note that includes each patient's subjective complaints, the objective information that you recorded, the physical agent that was applied and the manner of application, the response to the applied physical agent, and your assessment.

Laboratory Questions

1. What is the potential advantage of having the stimulation with IFC be capable of "moving"?

2. List three advantages and three disadvantages for IFC.

3. If the IFC device had carrier frequencies of 2000 Hz and 4000 Hz, how would you decide which would be more appropriate to use, or *would* one carrier be more appropriate than another?

4. What do you think would happen if you applied IFC to the lateral epicondyle and your patient changed the position of the elbow after you left the treatment area? (Try it and see!) (Also try elbow flexion with supination and pronation, and elbow extension with both supination and pronation.)

5. If your goal involved the reduction of pain and inflammation deep within the knee, what would be the optimal position for the patient and the electrodes for IFC?

6. If you do not cross the channels of the two generators from an IFC unit, are you producing IFC? Why or why not?

7. Why would the following electrode placement setup be considered contraindicated for any patient: one electrode on the superior aspect of the upper trapezius and the other electrode on the opposite side latissimus dorsi, with both channels crisscrossing the back?

8. Why would administration of ultrasound and frequency-difference IFC *not* be a good idea if the transducer served as one of the electrodes?

9. What would be the potential advantages for full-field IFC as opposed to frequency-difference IFC? Full-field IFC premodulates the carrier so that it is pulse-burst from the stimulator. There is no numbness underneath the electrodes as there is with frequency-difference IFC.

10. What would be the potential advantages for frequency-difference IFC as opposed to full-field IFC?

Electrical Stimulation Devices
(Knowing Whether the Equipment You Have Will Do What You Want It to Do)

Purpose

This laboratory exercise focuses on the devices themselves as tools to accomplish therapeutic treatment goals. Each of the previous laboratory exercises with electrical stimulation presented parameters to accomplish goals as a way of introducing the student to the device. Now the focus will be specifically on the goal, and how to make the stimulator do what you want it to do, or how to determine whether or not it is capable of doing what you want it to do. (Referring to previous laboratory exercises will be helpful.)

Objectives

- To translate terminology into the application of electrical stimulation for the accomplishment of therapeutic treatment goals
- To familiarize the student with the specification sheets of electrical stimulation devices
- To translate technical information into potential for therapeutic goal accomplishment

Equipment

various electrical stimulation units

electrodes and lead wires for each of the units

product specification sheets for electrical stimulation units

advertisements for electrical stimulation devices

Laboratory Exercises and Questions

1. Treatment goals for electrical stimulation include pain reduction, edema reduction, muscle strengthening, muscle reeducation, and muscle spasm reduction.
2. Select one of the stimulators, and identify what treatment goals could be accomplished with the unit based on the parameters that are available for that unit.
   a. Pain reduction?

   b. Edema reduction?

   c. Muscle strengthening?

   d. Muscle reeducation?

   e. Muscle spasm reduction?

3. Identify what treatment goals could not be accomplished with this stimulator. Why couldn't these goals be accomplished?

4. Select another electrical stimulation unit, and repeat steps 2 and 3.
    a. What are the common parameters for an electrical stimulator to be able to produce a muscle contraction in an innervated muscle?

    b. What parameters are necessary for the unit to be able to accomplish edema reduction or muscle strengthening?

    c. What are the necessary parameters for the unit to be able to accomplish sensory analgesia?

5. Review the mock specification sheets that follow, and indicate what each of the units could be used for (based on the available information in the specifications).

Excellence in stimulation	
Frequency:	0.1–1000 pps
Pulse duration:	50 μsec up to 2 sec
Intensity:	up to 1 mA
Channels:	2, 4, 6, or 8 independent channels
ON/OFF:	20-, 30-, 40-minute ON times
Ramps:	0.1 to 1 second up and down
Superb stimulator	
Frequency:	pain, edema, spasm
Pulse duration:	comfortable
Intensity:	sufficient for excellent pain relief
Channels:	1 or 2
ON/OFF:	unit beeps three short times to indicate end of treatment
Ramps:	no uncomfortable surging
Sensational stimulation	
Frequency:	1–250 pps (2500 Hz or 5000 Hz carrier frequency)
Pulse duration:	100–200 μsec (burst durations will vary)
Intensity:	up to 200 mA, 2 kΩ load tested
Channels:	1, 2, or 4 channels with independent current generators
ON/OFF:	4/4, 10/10, 10/50, or adjustable from continuous to independent times
Ramps:	independent ON/OFF ramps from 0.1 to 5 seconds
Creative currents	
Frequency:	1–120 pps
Pulse duration:	fixed at 50 μsec
Intensity:	1–500 Volts
Channels:	1 bifurcated lead channel
Ramps:	not applicable
Waveform:	twin spike, no net DC, polarity adjustable ±

6. Review the specification sheets and advertising materials describing electrical stimulation devices. Determine what each of the devices is capable of performing.
   a. What additional information, if any, would you need to make this determination?

   b. What was the terminology that was used in materials presented?

   c. Was the information clear?

   d. Would you be able to determine what the device could be used for if you were not able to speak with anyone about the device?

7. Design a stimulator that could be used for all therapeutic applications.
   a. What would you like to see it be able to do, and how would you make sure that it could do what you wanted it to do?

PATIENT SCENARIOS

Case Study A

It is late in the afternoon, and several patients are being treated with electrical stimulation units (as described in step 5). You are in search of a stimulator to accomplish muscle spasm reduction. All of the units except the "creative currents" unit are already being used. What would be the most appropriate course of action for you to take?

Case Study B

Brian, an Olympic pole vaulter, is being treated in your clinic for a tear to his hamstrings. Which of the units mentioned in step 5, if any, could be used for pain relief? Which of the units from step 5 could be used for muscle pumping to increase the nutrients into the medialis? Which of the units could be used for tissue healing?

Case Study C

Jane is an occupational therapist who has been referred to the physical therapy department for treatment of her painful edematous ankles. She is now in the end of her second trimester with twins. What potential treatment options do you have for her with stimulators mentioned in step 5?

Case Study D

Susan is an athletic trainer for the local community college women's field hockey team. She spends a great deal of time kneeling while taping the ankles of the team members. She fell down on her knees and has now been diagnosed with chondromalcia of the patella in both knees. There is marked weakness of the vastus medialis, edema superior to the patella, and a palpable painful crepitous in both knees when descending stairs.

The treatment goals include pain relief, edema reduction, and muscle strengthening.

A salesman comes into the physical therapy department that day and presents an inservice on a new stimulator. On further discussion, he makes the claim that his stimulator can treat all symptoms at the same time. What is wrong with this statement? What would you need to treat this patient and his symptoms?

DOCUMENTATION

Select two of the "patients" that you applied modalities to during the laboratory exercise, and write a progress note that includes each patient's subjective complaints, the objective information that you recorded, the physical agent that was applied, and the manner of application, the response to the applied physical agent, and your assessment.

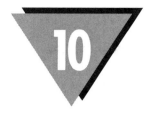

Hydrotherapy

Hydrotherapy is one of the fastest-growing applications of a physical agent modality in physical therapy practice today. It is not just the application of water in a therapeutic treatment tank, referred to as the *whirlpool*. Hydrotherapy encompasses the application of water to accomplish a therapeutic treatment goal. This is now commonly accomplished via the use of therapeutic pools that may be inside or outside the typical treatment environment, as well as the use of whirlpools in the clinical environment.

Purpose

This laboratory exercise is designed to familiarize the student with a wide variety of potential application techniques for water to accomplish therapeutic treatment goals. This modality is referred to as *hydrotherapy*.

Throughout this laboratory exercise, students will be instructed to apply or experience different forms of hydrotherapy that are commonly used in the clinic today. Questions will accompany each of the exercises. These questions are intended to help the student learn how to incorporate the use of hydrotherapy in clinical practice for the accomplishment of clinical treatment goals.

Objectives

- To demonstrate the physical principles of water through the use of guided laboratory activities
- To provide the student with a variety of experiences with therapeutic hydrotherapy
- To familiarize the student with the components of a therapeutic whirlpool
- To familiarize the student with the operation, care, and cleaning of the turbine and other components of a clinical whirlpool
- To familiarize the student with the difficulties in using whirlpools for medical patients, despite the potential advantages
- To provide the student with activities that will help to differentiate between the advantages and disadvantages of water versus "land" exercise programs
- To provide the student with the opportunity to learn about the benefits of buoyancy in therapeutic exercise programs

Equipment

towels	access to a therapeutic pool
various whirlpool tanks: Hi Boy, Low Boy, extremity tank, Hubbard tank	paddles (aquatic exercise devices)
	stethoscope and sphygmomonometer
bathing suits or tee shirts and shorts	

Precautions

healing wounds with granulation tissue
edematous extremities
sensitivity or allergies to additives in the water

Contraindications

split-thickness skin grafts prior to 3–5 days
full-thickness skin grafts prior to 7–10 days
full-body immersion when the vital capacity of the patient is less than 1500 mL

LABORATORY EXERCISES

Therapeutic Whirlpools

EQUIPMENT

1. Identify and name each piece of hydrotherapy equipment featured in Figure 10–1.

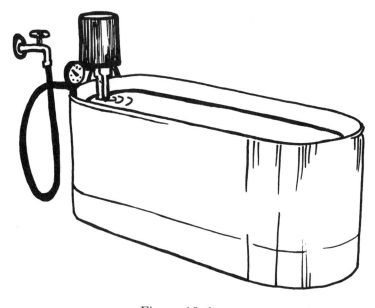

Figure 10–1

a. Find the turbine on the whirlpool.
b. Find the aeration adjustment on the turbine, and locate the breather opening(s). Indicate them on the illustration.

c. Determine how much water each tank holds, and list the amounts. Where did you find the information?
    • Hi Boy

    • Low Boy

    • Extremity tank

d. List the areas of the body that could be treated in each tank:
    • Hi Boy

    • Low Boy

    • Extremity tank

e. Fill and empty the tanks, recording the time to fill and your technique for filling the tank to maintain the water at 104°F.
    • Hi Boy

    • Low Boy (while it is full, perform the activities listed in Applications)

    • Extremity tank (while it is full, perform the activities listed in Applications)

APPLICATIONS

Low Boy

Perform the following activities:
1. Transfer a patient into the Low Boy from a wheelchair. He or she is non–weight bearing (NWB) on the left lower extremity (LLE). (The patient has no significant past medical history [PMH].)
    a. What planning is required in order for you to accomplish this task safely?

    b. What do you need to know about the patient *before* you transfer the patient into the tank?

    c. Of what significance is the water level in the tank prior to transferring the patient into the tank?

d. What transfer aids, if any, did you use?

e. Describe the sequence for the transfer and any difficulties that you may have had with the transfer, outlining how you would approach it the next time.

2. Adjust the patient's position so that he or she is long-sitting in the Low Boy. Support the patient's back and arms so that no excess pressure is exerted on them. (A towel roll may be used to cushion the extremities from the edges of the tank.)
   a. Turn on the turbine, and adjust it so that the turbulence is directed at a 45° angle to the left side of the tank. What does the patient report? Where does the patient feel the agitation?

   b. Decrease the amount of air that flows into the turbine. How does this change the sensation that the patient has reported?

   c. Increase the amount of air flow to maximum. How does the sensation that the patient feels change, if at all?

   d. Adjust the turbine so that it is pointing directly at the patient. What is the patient's response to the adjustment?

   e. After 5 minutes of submersion and adjustments to the turbine air flow, recheck the water temperature. Has it changed? If yes, why?

3. Prepare your patient to be transferred out of the tank and back into the wheel-chair. List the steps that you need to perform.

4. How would you document what you just did?

5. Repeat the transfers in and out of the Low Boy until you are comfortable with what you will need to consider to assure patient and personal safety.

Extremity Tank

Perform the following activities:
1. Position your patient to have the right foot treated in the extremity tank.
   a. What considerations do you need to make?

2. You will need to adjust the turbine to perform nonspecific débridement to a fragile calcaneal ulcer.
   a. What considerations do you need to make, and how would you adjust the turbine?

b. What things would change if the patient were being treated for an acute ankle sprain?

c. Describe some of the problems that you encountered and how you addressed them.

Extremity Tank

Perform the following activities:
1. Position your patient to have the left elbow treated in the extremity tank.
   a. What consideration do you need to make (body mechanics, and so forth)?

Hubbard Tank

Perform the following activities:
1. Observe and then demonstrate the use of the Hubbard tank and its lift by transferring one of your classmates into the tank.
2. Discuss appropriate instructions for the patient, as well as indications, contraindications, and precautions for the use of the Hubbard tank itself and for the lift.

Empty and clean each of the tanks that you used!

1. What is the procedure for cleaning the whirlpools?

2. Where did you find the information for cleaning the tanks?

3. What is the procedure for cleaning the turbines?

4. Why do the turbines need to run while cleaning?

TREATMENT CONSIDERATIONS

Discuss the following potential patients for hydrotherapy, considering the indications and potential benefits of hydrotherapy for each of the conditions described. Determine the appropriate equipment, water temperatures, whether to use agitation, and whether hydrotherapy would be indicated for the patients described.

Case Study A

Mrs. Heal is an 80-year-old slender woman with a L calcaneal decubitus ulcer. She has a PMH of diabetes.

Hydrotherapy indicated? _____Yes _____No
Equipment

Water temperature

Agitation used

Comments

Case Study B

John Klutz is a 25-year-old man with s/p ORIF of the R ankle and spasm of the right calf musculature. His incision is well healed, and he is PWB on the R leg with crutches. His ROM in dorsiflexion and plantarflexion are limited.

Hydrotherapy indicated? _____Yes _____No
Equipment

Water temperature

Agitation used

Comments

Case Study C

Betty Shelhouse is a 60-year-old woman with s/p RLE long-leg cast removal. She lives alone in a first-floor condominium and has been ambulating NWB on the R leg with a walker. She has good strength throughout upper and lower extremities. She is anxious to resume her schedule, which included aerobics and bicycling.

Hydrotherapy indicated? _____Yes _____No
Equipment

Water temperature

Agitation used

Comments

Case Study D

Mike Hacker is a 35-year-old man who experienced a traumatic amputation of his LUE above the elbow. The injury occurred 8 weeks ago. He is anxious to resume working. His amputation scar is well healed, and he will be fitted with a prosthesis as soon as the stump is toughened up. His UE strength is poor, and he fatigues easily since the injury. He has inquired about a possible home program.

Hydrotherapy indicated? _____Yes _____No
Equipment

Water temperature

Agitation used

Comments

Case Study E

Marty Nealy is a 55-year-old woman who is now s/p 8 weeks for a below-the-knee amputation of the RLE secondary to insensate ulcerations as a result of diabetes. She is now anxious to be fitted for a prosthesis and to begin ambulation activities. Her incision is well healed, and she has no other significant PMH.

Hydrotherapy indicated? _____Yes _____No
Equipment

Water temperature

Agitation used

Comments

Case Study F

Mary Tomlin is a 68-year-old obese woman with severe osteoporosis of the hip bilaterally. She was referred to the physical therapy department after a fall that resulted in a compound fracture of the left femur. The fracture has now healed. Goals include increasing strength and promoting weight bearing to prevent further bone loss.

Hydrotherapy indicated? _____Yes _____No
Equipment

Water temperature

Agitation used

Comments

Case Study G

Bill Back is a 45-year-old man with s/p 8 weeks lumbar laminectomy with bilateral muscle guarding of the paraspinal musculature. He is working as an architect and is limited in all spinal movement because of this muscle guarding. He formerly was very active as a triathelete. He needs mobility and aerobic exercises that will allow the paraspinal muscles to relax.

Hydrotherapy indicated? _____Yes _____No
Equipment

Water temperature

Agitation used

Comments

Case Study H

Brian Young is a 22-year-old man with an acute sprain (3 days ago) of the anterior talofibular ligament. His ankle is edematous but pain-free. His ankle ROM is limited in all directions by muscle guarding. He is anxious to return to work as a mail carrier.

Hydrotherapy indicated? _____Yes _____No
Equipment

Water temperature

Agitation used

Comments

Case Study I

Sharon Yale is a 68-year-old woman with s/p R radical mastectomy, with decreased shoulder ROM in all directions. Her incisions are well healed, and she is anxious to resume as much activity as possible. She had been an aerobics instructor for a senior citizen center.

Hydrotherapy indicated? _____Yes _____No
Equipment

Water temperature

Agitation used

Comments

Case Study J

Jim Lennos is a 45-year-old man who had an arthroscopic meniscectomy of the left knee 4 weeks ago. His incision is well healed, and he is now FWB on the L leg. He is complaining of weakness and that his knee "gives out" when he descends stairs.

Hydrotherapy indicated? _____Yes _____No
Equipment

Water temperature

Agitation used

Comments

Therapeutic Aquatic Pools

1. Record your vital signs:

HR: _____BP:_____Resp: _____(per minute)

    a. What is the temperature of the pool?

    b. What is the time when you entered the pool?

2. You will be *in* a therapeutic pool for the following activities. It is suggested that you appoint a reader/recorder to read and record your responses from the laboratory while you are in the water.

RESISTANCE

1. Walk in water that is knee deep, waist deep, and shoulder deep. What difference does the depth make in your ease of movement?

2. Walk forward in shoulder-depth water, and stop quickly. What happens? Why?

3. Try to run in the water. What happens?

4. Stand in shoulder-depth water, and slowly abduct your right shoulder horizontally, stopping at 45°.
    a. Does your arm have a tendency to move or stop in this position?

b. Would this be a gravity-assisted position on land?

c. How would you describe the position in the water (buoyancy resisted or assisted)?

5. What could you do to increase the amount of resistance to movement that you encounter in the water? Try it. Does it work?

a. If a patient tried your technique to increase the resistance, would there be any additional considerations? If yes, what would they be?

6. What happens when you push your hands down to your sides (with pronated forearms) from the surface of the water?

a. What happens when you repeat this with your forearms in a neutral position? Why?

7. "Float" in the water.
   a. What areas of your body are below the surface of the water, and why?

b. What happens when you extend your hip?

c. What exercise or motion would this position be providing buoyancy assistance for and buoyancy resistance for?

8. Come out of the pool, and record the following:
   a. Vital signs:

HR: _____BP:_____Resp: _____(per minute)

b. Pool temperature:

c. Time you exited the pool:

d. How long were you in the pool?

e. How if at all did your vital signs change? Why or why not?

f. Based on the changes that you saw in your vital signs or in those of your classmates, what impact would similar changes have on patients who were involved in aquatic pool programs?

PATIENT SCENARIOS

Go back and address each of the patients described in the first section of this laboratory under Treatment Considerations, and describe who would potentially benefit from an aquatic pool program. Describe the program that you think would be most beneficial for each of them.

DOCUMENTATION

The purpose of documentation is to provide an accurate record of the treatment rendered. It should contain elements of the treatment technique and specific details of its application if its application was performed in any unusual and uncustomary manner. It should also provide an assessment of the patient's response to the treatment intervention.

Hydrotherapy treatments should be documented indicating the type of hydrotherapy intervention used: whirlpool or aquatic pool. For whirlpools, documentation should also indicate the temperature of the water, whether agitation was used, and whether any additives were used in the water. For aquatic pools, temperature, depth of immersion, treatment time, and any special equipment that was used should be documented. Any significant changes in the vital signs of the patient should also be recorded, along with an assessment and plan based on these changes.

Select two of the "patients" that you applied modalities to during the laboratory exercise, and write a progress note that includes the patient's subjective complaints, objective information that you recorded, the physical agent that was applied, the manner of application, the response to the applied physical agent, and your assessment.

Laboratory Questions

1. Approximately how long should you allow for the preparation of a whirlpool?

2. What additional considerations are there for positioning and body mechanics with Hi-Boy and Low-Boy whirlpools?

3. Describe the benefits of nonspecific débridement.

4. Describe the potential harm that a turbine can cause to a healing ulcer and how the harm could be prevented.

5. If your patient has been diagnosed with a spinal cord injury that is now stable at T4, what potential reasons would there be to have the patient participate in an aquatic pool program?

6. What additional benefits are derived from deep-water activities in an aquatic pool that are not possible in land exercises?

7. Other than ROM in a buoyancy-assisted environment, what are the benefits of aquatic therapy for postmastectomy patients?

8. Describe how flotation devices could be used to increase the level of resistance for an exercise program.

Therapeutic Uses of Light
Actinotherapy

Purpose

This laboratory exercise involves the use of two different forms of light that induce either chemical reactions or thermal responses in the treated tissue. You will be comparing and contrasting the two forms of light.

Objectives

- To provide the student with the opportunity to experience both infrared (IR) and UV radiation
- To provide the student with the opportunity to solve patient positioning and draping problems for the application of IR and UV radiation
- To familiarize students with the importance of the use of protective eye wear when using UV radiation
- To provide the students with the opportunity to perform a minimal erythema dose (MED) for UV radiation

Equipment

towels

UV lamp

timer (seconds)

protective goggles for UV
    exposure

IR lamp

tape measure

materials to make a test strip for an MED

Precautions

burned skin (first degree)

freckled skin

minor scars that are healed

Contraindications

Infrared radiation:

over second- or third-degree
  burned skin

over insensate areas

over the gonads

over the eyes

in the presence of metal in the
  treatment area

Ultraviolet radiation:

in patients diagnosed with lupus
  erythematosus, pellagra

in patients who are taking
  photosensitive medications

over the eyes

over the gonads

in patients with active tuberculosis

in patients with acute
  diabetes or fever

LABORATORY EXERCISES

Ultraviolet Radiation

You may answer the following questions based on your knowledge of the application of UV from the lecture and your reading assignments. You should be able to predict most of the responses and remedies. You may need to administer a timed exposure to establish what an MED would be equivalent to for a given patient. Some of the newer equipment has predetermined dosage levels and shielding devices built into the apparatus.

For this exercise, you will be performing an MED for UV radiation.

1. Select two classmates/patients for UV MED determination. One should have fairer skin than the other. There should be no other distinguishing differences between the two patients (for example, no scars or wounds).

2. Position your patients so that the medial aspect of their distal upper extremity is exposed. The rest of the patients' bodies should be draped, and the patients should wear protective goggles. Anyone who is facing the UV lamp should also wear protective goggles appropriate for the specific wavelength of the lamp.

3. Prepare a testing board with four square openings in it. Each opening should measure $\frac{1}{4} \times \frac{1}{4}$ inch and be spaced linearly about $\frac{1}{2}$ inch apart.

4. Secure the testing board to your patient's forearm, the drape your patient again so that none of the openings are exposed.

5. Position the lamp so that it is both 30 inches from the patient and perpendicular to the area to be exposed.

6. Allow the lamp to warm up prior to opening up the doors to the bulb. While the lamp is warming up, have all who face the lamp put on protective eye wear.

7. Once the lamp is ready, open it, and reveal the top opening on your patient's forearm for 120 seconds.

8. Continue to monitor the time, and uncover the second opening for another 30 seconds.

9. Continue to monitor the time, and uncover the third opening for another 30 seconds.

10. Continue to monitor the time, and uncover the fourth opening for another 30 seconds.

11. Close the lamp, turn it OFF, and remove it from the treatment area. Undrape your patients, and inspect the skin. There were a total of four areas exposed to the UV radiation, each for slightly different amounts of time.
12. Observe your patients over the next 12, 24, and 36 hours. Note which, if any, of the four openings on their forearms become darker in appearance.

Infrared Radiation

Read through the following description of an IR treatment setup, and answer the questions based on your understanding of how IR works. If you have time and the appropriate equipment, you may setup this patient.
1. Select a classmate/patient to be treated for cervical pain and muscle spasm.
2. Observe the patient's skin in the cervical region. Are there any remarkable scars or lesions; is the skin tanned, freckled, or particularly hairy; does the skin have any other abnormalities?

3. Position your patient so that he or she is supported and comfortable.
4. Place the IR lamp so that it is 90 cm from the patient, and turn it on. The lamp should be perpendicular to the patient's skin. Ask the patient to describe the sensation under the lamp after 5 minutes and after 10 minutes.

5. Observe the skin under the lamp, noting any changes that you observe.

6. Now repeat the setup with another patient. This time, place the lamp 45 cm from the patient. What does the patient report after 5 minutes? After 10 minutes?

DOCUMENTATION

Documentation for both UV and IR radiation should include the time of exposure, the treatment area, the patient's response to the exposure, and the manufacturer of the lamp, if there is more than one lamp in the department.

Select two of the "patients" that you applied modalities to during the lab exercise, and write a progress note that includes each patient's subjective complaints, the objective information that you recorded, the physical agent that was applied and the manner of application, the response to the applied physical agent, and your assessment.

LABORATORY QUESTIONS

1. Which patient(s) felt something from the treatment? Why?

2. Were there any changes in the appearance of the patient's skin immediately after treatment with either of the two modalities? If yes, what? If no, why not?

3. Which patient, if any, felt warmth? When?

4. Why did the lamps need to be placed perpendicular to the patient?

5. What would happen to the dosage if the angle between the UV lamp and the patient was less than 90°?

6. When would you select IR radiation as a form of superficial heat treatment for a patient?

7. If a patient complained of too much heat from the IR lamp, what could be done to remedy this?

8. Why would it be appropriate to observe the skin 12–36 hours after exposure to UV? What would you be looking for?

9. What advantages are there to light as a therapeutic modality?

10. What disadvantages are there to light as a therapeutic modality?

11. Why were lupus and photosensitive medications considered contraindications for patients to receive UV?

12. In your opinion, why are UV and IR lamps not commonly used?

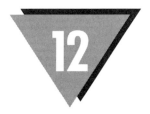

Passive Motion Devices for Soft Tissue Management
Traction

Purpose

This laboratory exercise is designed to demonstrate the principles of therapeutic traction currently practiced in clinical environments. Students will become familiar with the treatment goals, positioning, apparatus, and techniques used. Students will have the opportunity to administer and receive various forms of traction. Students will learn the importance of proper positioning of the patient, the device, and the individual applying the traction. They will also learn what to document and how important appropriate patient instruction is to treatment success.

Objectives

- To familiarize the student with the operation of mechanical traction equipment devices
- To familiarize the student with the importance of proper patient positioning during traction
- To familiarize the student with the importance of relaxation as a technique to decrease the stresses on postural muscles so that a traction force may be successfully applied
- To provide the student with the opportunity to experience various types of traction
- To familiarize the student with the proper application of supports, belts, and straps to accomplish mechanical traction
- To provide the student with the opportunity to stabilize an extremity while manual traction is being applied

Equipment

mechanical traction unit (with manual)	adhesive tape	pillows
empty plastic gallon milk bottle	cervical traction head halter	a string "plumb bob"
belts and straps for traction unit	goniometer towels foot stool	a protractor (optional) Saunders Cervical Traction appliance

Precautions

joint hypermobility
cardiac or respiratory insufficiency
pregnancy (inversion traction)
acute inflammation

temporomandibular joint dysfunction
  (cervical claustrophobia
  traction)

Contraindications

spinal infections that could be spread
  through the use of traction
rheumatoid arthritis
osteoporosis

spinal cancers
spinal cord pressure (secondary to
  central disk herniation)
fused spine (surgical or congenital)

LABORATORY EXERCISES

Patient Positioning

SUPINE

1. Have one of your classmates lie supine on a plinth without any pillows. Position your classmate so that there is a straight line along midline, bisecting the right and left sides.
   a. What were your points of reference to determine that your patient was "straight"?

   b. Is your patient comfortable?

   c. What is the position of the lumbar spine (lordosis or not)?

   d. What is the position of the cervical spine?

2. Position your classmate so that he or she has a flat lordosis and a neutral cervical lordosis.
   a. Describe what you needed to do to accomplish this.

   b. Is your patient comfortable in this position?

   c. Is your patient still straight with a bisecting midline?

   d. How long does it take to position the patient so that he or she is positioned with both a flat lordosis and a neutral cervical spine?

3. Grasp the humerus of your classmate superior to the distal shaft, so that you can apply gross distraction/traction to the right upper extremity.
   a. What happens to the alignment of your patient?

   b. How much traction force did it take for the alignment to shift?

4. Reposition your classmate. This time, have another classmate stabilize the acromion and trunk while you distract the humerus.
   a. What happens to the alignment of your patient?

   b. How much traction force did it take for the alignment to shift this time?

   c. What purpose would stabilization serve when applying traction?

5. Arrange the straps for lumbar traction so that the thoracic strap is at the top of a plinth and the lumbar strap is below it on the plinth so that when the patient lies supine on the plinth, the straps will be underneath. Be careful to position your patient so that midline for the straps aligns with midline for the patient. Secure the straps so that the patient can still breathe, but tighten them enough so that when a traction force is applied, the straps will not slip.

   Now support the knees of the patient in about 90° of flexion by placing a footstool underneath the lower legs. Support the cervical spine in a neutral position.
   a. What happens to the alignment of the patient whenever you tighten a strap or place a pillow under the cervical spine or a footstool under the legs?

   b. How does your patient feel in this position and equipment?

   Attach the straps to the spreader bar and then to the traction unit. Recheck patient alignment. The patient's midline should line up with the center pull from the traction straps.
   c. How long did it take for you to set up the patient so that the patient was aligned and supported appropriately?

d. What do you think the potential consequences would be if the alignment was not straight and the traction force was applied?

SITTING

1. Have one of your classmates sit in a chair that has a straight back (armrests optional). The classmate should be positioned so that the feet are flat and firmly touching the floor and he or she has an erect posture with a straight line running from the tragus of the ear through the acromion process, the spine, and the greater trochanter.

   a. Describe what you needed to do to accomplish this positioning.

   b. What tools did you use to assess the position?

   c. Is your patient comfortable in this position?

   d. How long did it take to accomplish this position?

   e. While you were recording your answers, did your patient shift position? If yes, how?

f. If your goal was to relieve the pressure of the head on the cervical spine created by gravity, where would the "pull" or "line of pull" need to come?

g. How would you stabilize the rest of the body?

2. Select one of the cervical head halters, and inspect it. Determine which is the mandibular strap and which is the occipital strap. With your patient seated, place the halter on him or her.
    There should be two metal rings or half rings on the straps in between the mandibular and occipital straps. Hold onto both rings, one in each hand on each side of the head. Gently pull upward to take up the slack in the straps; do not try to relieve the weight of the head.
    a. If your goal were to relieve the weight of the head, what direction or angle would you need to have the traction pull toward? (Look at the cervical spine. The line of pull should be coming off of the occiput, not the mandible.)

    b. Why would it be important *not* to have the pull come from the mandible?

    c. How difficult is it to adjust the line of pull to accomplish an occipital pull? What do you need to do?

MOCK CERVICAL TRACTION SETUP

1. Fill the empty milk container with water and recap it, securing the cap with a ring of adhesive tape. This will be the "head" for this exercise. The handle of the milk bottle represents the posterior upper cervical spine, and it comes from the base of the occiput. The "cap" of the bottle is inferior to the chin of the mandible.

2. Place a ring of adhesive tape around the base of the occiput and around the entire head (bottle) so that it bisects the head just below the nose. The line of tape should be perpendicular to the seam on the bottle (Fig. 12–1).

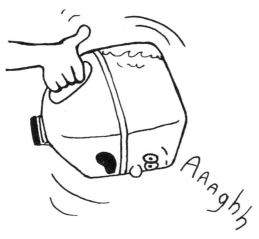

Figure 12–1

3. Place another line of tape on the anterior seam of the bottle. This will be an additional reference point for positioning.

4. You will note that handling a bottle that is full of water is not easy. The weight of the gallon container is approximately _____, which is actually less than the weight of the head.

5. You will also note that resting the bottle on the table so that the seam is facing up and aligned is not easy either. The human head is much the same. The patient will have a tendency to turn the head to one side to rest, as the head does not balance in neutral easily (Fig. 12–2).

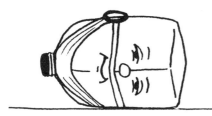

Figure 12–2

6. Apply a cervical halter to the bottle. Determine what angle the line of pull will need to be in order to relieve the weight of the head (Figs. 12–3 and 12–4).

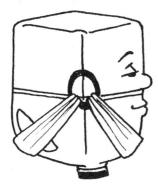

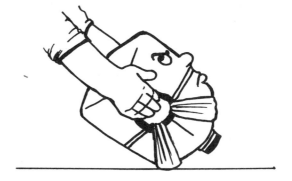

Figure 12–3

Figure 12–4

OBSERVATIONS AND QUESTIONS

1. Ask one of your laboratory instructors to demonstrate manual cervical traction with the patient in both a seated and a supine position.
   a. Which position appeared "easier" for the clinician? Why?

   b. Which position appeared more comfortable for the patient? Why?

2. Cervical traction is usually applied in the supine position.
   a. Why do you think that this would be true?

3. Ask one of the laboratory instructors to set up the Saunders Cervical Traction appliance, attaching it to a mechanical traction unit.
   a. Before a patient is positioned on the plinth, can you predict which position the appliance will place the cervical spine in?

   b. Inspect the appliance. What is the purpose of the small "sled" that the occiput rests on?

   c. Inspect the straps and supports for the appliance. What is the purpose for the temporal/frontal strap?

   d. How is the mandible "treated" with this appliance? (Is there any support for it or pull on it?)

4. If you were to give your seated cervical traction patient a magazine to "pass the time" while he or she was in traction, what happens to the positioning?

5. If you were to instruct a supine patient to "just get up" after a traction force had been applied and released, what would happen to the intradisk pressure?

6. Why would the position of the patient prior to the application of a traction force make a difference?

7. How much force would it take to overcome the weight of the head in the sitting position? In the supine position? In the supine position with the cervical appliance?

8. What happened to the pressure on the mandible when you tried to adjust the angle of pull to the occiput on the bottle?

9. The cervical spine has two individual curves. Of what significance would they be when applying cervical traction?

10. Which muscles maintain the normal cervical curves?

11. Which muscles tend to guard following a cervical strain, and what impact, if any, would muscle guarding in these muscles have on the curves in the cervical spine?

PATIENT SCENARIOS

Read through the patient scenarios, and determine the following:
- Whether or not traction would be indicated and your rationale for your response
- What the parameters for traction should be for the patient if traction is indicated
- How the patient should be positioned
- What type of straps would be used if you decide to use a mechanical form of traction
- Where the pull should be coming from for the applied traction force
- What additional considerations that there might be for a patient to be considered a good candidate for traction
- Whether or not the traction should be applied clinically or at home and why

Case Study A

If you were instructed to apply cervical traction for the reduction of cervical muscle pain and guarding for a patient who had unilateral guarding of the upper trapezius on the right, what if anything about the treatment setup would change?

Case Study B

Mr. Mason is a construction worker who injured his back while installing a steel grate to cover a drainage basin. His pain occurred after he let go of the grate and when he attempted to straighten up. He has radicular symptoms in the left leg. Would traction of some form be indicated? If yes, how? If not, why? What additional considerations might there be for this patient?

Case Study C

S. Smile was referred to the physical therapy department for cervical traction following an automobile accident in which her car was struck from behind. She has bilateral guarding in all cervical muscles. She recently underwent a mandibular reduction to correct horizontal alignment of her incisors. Her incisions are now well healed, and in the 8 weeks since the surgery, she had been steadily increasing the amount of vertical opening of her mandible until the automobile accident 2 weeks ago. What additional considerations are there for this patient? Would traction be contraindicated? Why or why not?

Case Study D

Steve W. has been referred to the physical therapy department by his physician for lumbar traction to relieve questionable lumbar radiculopathies that appear to be transient. Steve injured his back while working, and he has not returned to work yet. His complaints of pain and numbness vary. Some days, the paresthesia is located in the right foot, and other days, it is in the left foot. Traction was suggested to see if centralization of the pain was possible. There was no sign of fracture.

One day after traction, Steve returns to the clinic for another treatment. He states that his symptoms did subside following the traction. Today, his paresthesia is behind his left knee, but he also complains of pain in the right buttocks. When setting up the lumbar belts, you ask whether or not Steve needs to use the restroom prior to the traction. Steve declines and states that for some reason, he has not been able to urinate for about the last 12 hours. What course of action should you take? Why?

DOCUMENTATION

As with other modalities, it is important to document the treatment parameters used. You must document the following parameters:
- Patient position: supine, knees flexed or extended, prone, sitting, and so forth
- Line of pull: unilateral pull, central pull, and so forth
- Type of traction: mechanical, intermittent, sustained, manual
- Amount of force: pounds
- Duration: holding time, resting time
- Attachments: Saunders Cervical Traction, cervical halter, over-the-door home unit
- Total treatment time

It is also important to document the patient's initial complaint prior to the traction and his or her response to the traction. Traction is commonly applied to relieve radicular symptoms; you should indicate whether or not it accomplished the goal. Sometimes a patient will report a decrease in the symptoms during the traction but a return of the symptoms once the traction force is released. This should also be documented.

Select two of the "patients" that you applied modalities to during the laboratory exercise, and write a progress note that includes the patient's subjective complaints, objective information that you recorded, the physical agent that was applied, the manner of application, the response to the applied physical agent, and your assessment.

LABORATORY QUESTIONS

1. What was the significance of the gallon bottle for the mock traction setup?

2. Describe how your body mechanics might change if you were performing manual cervical traction while a patient was seated in a chair and while lying supine.

3. If cervical and lumbar traction are performed to relieve radiculopathies, what is the goal of appendicular manual traction?

4. Of what significance is the hand placement of the individual who is stabilizing a patient during a manual traction treatment?

Passive Motion Devices for Soft Tissue Management
Continuous Passive Motion

Continuous passive motion (CPM) devices have been used to improve joint mobility postoperatively. It is common for the devices to be applied immediately postoperatively. All health-care providers who will be interfacing with the patient need to be familiar with the operation of these devices.

Purpose

This laboratory focuses on the operation of an upper extremity and a lower extremity device. Students will be adjusting the range of motion (ROM), the speed, and the patient positioning to experience the sensations that a patient would experience.

Objectives

- To familiarize the student with the operation of CPM devices for the upper and the lower extremity
- To provide students with the opportunity to set up a CPM device on a classmate
- To provide students with the opportunity to solve patient positioning problems that arise with CPM devices
- To provide students with the opportunity to experience CPM for both an upper and a lower extremity

- To familiarize students with the necessary patient instructions to prevent possible injury or complication from the use of a CPM

Equipment

upper extremity CPM (and manual)   goniometer
lower extremity CPM (and manual)   sheepskin or other pressure-relieving cloth

Precautions

claustrophobia
external fixation devices

Contraindications

fused joints   hemophilia or blood-thinning
unstable fractures   medications
                                          renal failure

The Devices

1. Select one of the upper extremity CPM devices. Read through the manual, and identify the following:
   - Mechanism that moves the extremity
   - ROM-limiting device
   - Speed control settings
   - Supports to stabilize the extremity
   a. Which joint(s) is this particular device designed to be used for?

   b. How long after surgery should this device be applied?

   c. What are the most common applications for this device?

2. Select a classmate/patient to wear the CPM. Your patient is presently resting in the supine position. Apply the device so that the joint(s) move through all but the last 20° of motion at a slow speed.
   a. What problems do you encounter when setting up the device?

   b. What would be considered an optimal patient position for this device?

   c. Recheck the ROM on the device. Is it accurate?

   d. Approximately how long did it take you to set up the device?

3. Remove the device, and trade places with your patient. Repeat the setup as before.
   a. What problems did you encounter when setting up the device?

   b. Is your patient comfortable in the same positions that you were comfortable in? What might account for this?

c. Recheck the axis of the joint(s), and remeasure the ROM. Have they shifted? If so, how?

d. Approximately how long did it take you to set up the device?

4. Remove the device from your patient. Return the device, and select another CPM. Repeat the same steps. You should be trying an upper and a lower extremity device as both the patient and the clinician.

DOCUMENTATION

CPM devices have more than one manufacturer and more than one application. For this reason, it is important to document the manufacturer and model of the device. It is also important to document the ROM, speed, resting time, positioning, and amount of time that the device is to be left on the extremity. A copy of the instructions for operation of the device that were given to the patient should be attached to the patient's chart. These instructions should indicate who the patient is to contact if he or she has any questions about the device or its operation.

Select two of the "patients" that you applied modalities to during the laboratory exercise, and write a progress note that includes the patient's subjective complaints, objective information that you recorded, the physical agent that was applied, the manner of application, the response to the applied physical agent, and your assessment.

LABORATORY QUESTIONS

1. How difficult was it for you to set up the patient with the appropriate limitation in ROM? What made it difficult?

2. Was the setup time shorter after you had already set up the CPM once?

3. Which was harder to set up: the upper extremity or the lower extremity CPM? Why?

4. Which device was more uncomfortable when it was on: the upper or the lower extremity device? Were you able to remedy the discomfort? Why or why not?

5. What would you instruct a patient about that was not covered in the instructions that came with the device?

6. What suggestions (if any) would you make to the manufacturer of the CPM so that it would be easier for a patient to use?

7. Of what significance would noncompliance with the use of the device be?

Edema Management
Intermittent Compression as a Therapeutic Tool

There are multiple causes of edema, and it represents a complex problem for both the patient and the clinician. You will be practicing assessment techniques for edema, because without accurate measurement of the edema, it would be impossible to determine whether the technique used proved effective.

Purpose

This laboratory focuses on the therapeutic techniques for the management of edema. Part of the laboratory also focuses on the appropriate use of intermittent compression devices as a treatment modality for edema management.

Objectives

- To familiarize the student with a wide variety of edema assessment techniques
- To provide the student with the opportunity to practice edema assessment
- To practice using a tape measure and a volumeter
- To practice measurement of edema
- To practice setting up an intermittent compression device
- To gain familiarity with intermittent compression devices
- To practice monitoring pedal, popliteal, and radial pulses

Equipment

vinyl tape measure,
   goniometer
upper extremity volumeter
foot volumeter
catch basin for water
large graduated cylinder

thermometer
marking pen
sphygmomanometer
   and stethoscope
intermittent
   compression device

upper and
   lower extremity
   appliances for
   compression device
disposable stockinet

Precautions

patients taking diuretics (may need more frequent rest periods for voiding)
decreased cognitive ability of the patient

Contraindications

acute pulmonary edema
acute trauma
acute localized infection (in the
   treatment area)

congestive heart failure
acute deep vein thrombosis
acute unstable fracture

LABORATORY EXERCISES

Edema Assessment with a Tape Measure

1. Select two classmates/patients who have different body sizes. You will be taking circumferential measurements of their right and left upper extremities. Position your patients so that they are supine with the extremity to be measured first and make sure that the extremity is elevated and supported. (In order for you to measure the extremity, you will need to support both the distal and proximal aspects.)
2. Clean your tape measure with alcohol. Place a mark on the medial aspect of the forearm at the level of the styloid process of the ulna. Place another mark at the bicepital crease of the elbow.
3. Using the tape measure, place a mark on the skin every 1½ inches moving proximally to the axilla from the elbow and distally every 1½ inches to the wrist. (A small mark is preferred as some inks may cause allergic reactions or injure fragile skin.)
   a. Record your measurements on the chart in Figure 14–1.
   b. Have another one of your classmates perform the same measurements, and compare his or her measurements to those that you recorded.

Upper Extremity Measurements

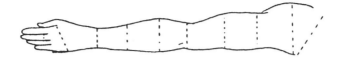

Date																			
Side																			
wrist																			
6" b.e.																			
4.5" b																			
3" be																			
1.5"																			
elbow																			
1.5"ae																			
3" ae																			
4.5"																			
6" a.e.																			

Figure 14–1

4. Switch places with your patients, and repeat the process of measurement. Compare your findings.

Edema Assessment with a Volumeter

1. Select two classmates/patients who will have the volume of their foot and ankle assessed through use of a volumeter.
2. Fill the volumeter with water to the starting line. The water should be warm (above 99°F, 37°C), and the temperature of the water should be recorded.
3. Inspect the foot to be immersed. Make sure that it is clean and that there are no open lesions.
4. Position the catch basin so that it is below the spout of the volumeter.
5. Have your patient stand so that the foot is flat on the bottom of the volumeter. Water will flow out the spout into the basin (Fig. 14–2).
   a. Record the volume of water displaced by using the graduated cylinder.

6. Empty the water, clean the volumeter, and refill it. Repeat these steps, but this time, use cold water (about 40°F, 4°C)
   a. Record your measurements and observations.

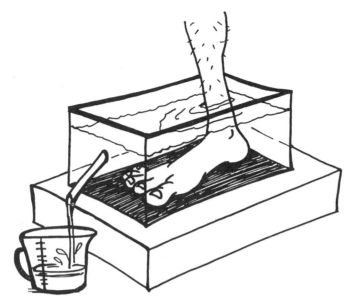

Figure 14–2

Intermittent Compression Devices

1. Read the instruction manual for the device. Locate the controls on the device that will adjust the inflation pressure, the deflation pressure, ON/OFF times, and treatment time. Select a classmate/patient for intermittent compression to the lower extremity.
2. Position and drape your patient so that he or she will be comfortable. Inspect the extremity for open lesions, hematomas, and so forth.
3. Measure the extremity from the ankle to about 9 inches proximal to the knee using the same technique as for the upper extremity.
   a. Record your measurements in a chart.

4. Monitor the pedal and popliteal pulses.
   a. Obtain and record the resting heart rate and blood pressure.

5. Apply a stockinet to the extremity. (Make sure that there are no folds or creases.)
6. Apply the lower extremity appliance. Recheck the patient's positioning so that the leg is elevated and supported.
7. Check the inflation and deflation pressures on the device. Set the inflation pressure to 50 mmHg and the deflation pressure to 20 mmHg.
8. Set the ON time to 20 seconds and OFF time to 6 seconds. (If you cannot individually set these parameters or the device has preset parameters, select the preset that is closest to this ratio and record your settings.)
9. Start the device. Stay until the inflation is complete, and then until the device has gone through two complete cycles. Let the device run for 15 minutes. (Check your patient to make sure that he or she is comfortable.)

10. Once the time is up, deflate, remove the appliance, remove the stockinet, and quickly remeasure the extremity. Record your findings and observations.

11. Repeat this exercise so that other classmates have the opportunity to feel the compression appliance as it inflates and deflates.

PATIENT SCENARIOS

Read through the patient scenarios, and determine the following:
- Whether or not intermittent compression would be indicated
- If you decided that it was not indicated due to a lack of information, what additional information you would need to know
- If indicated, what a realistic expectation of the treatment would be
- If indicated, how it would be applied:
    Patient position
    Patient instruction
    Additional considerations for the patient
- How you will assess whether or not your parameter selections were appropriate
- When intermittent compression would be contraindicated
- When edema assessment techniques should be employed
- Which edema assessment technique would be the most appropriate

Case Study A

Mike is a roofer who has been referred to the physical therapy department for an injury to his left ankle that was the result of his falling off a ladder. His ankle is now edematous, particularly anterior to the lateral malleolus. Mike fell 3 weeks ago, but he didn't seek medical attention until now because he didn't want to miss work. There were no fractures noted by the physician. Mike has a long history of ankle sprains and strains, approximately one per year for the past 10 years. Other than being diabetic, he has no other significant medical history. His chief complaint is that he is unable to wear his work boots because of the swelling. He has no complaints of pain.

Case Study B

Karen is a legal secretary who was referred to the physical therapy department for lymphedema secondary to a radical mastectomy of the left breast. Karen was diagnosed with breast cancer approximately 6 months ago. Since the surgery, she has had bouts of depression and has been unable to work. She is now undergoing chemotherapy, and her physician has assured her that there were no signs of active cancer in the surrounding tissues. Her left arm is so edematous that she has difficulty lifting it, which makes work impossible for her now.

Case Study C

Inga is a hairdresser who has been having a great deal of difficulty with fluid retention in both legs. She is on her feet all day and rarely has a chance to sit down. In addition, she is now 5 months pregnant with her first child. Inga has been referred to the physical therapy department for edema reduction. She has no significant medical history.

Case Study D

Keith is a college student who is returning to school after retiring from another career. He has three grown children who live at home with him and his wife. One of his daughters is pregnant and has been having a difficult time with the pregnancy. Keith is obese and has a classic "type A personality." So far his GPA is a 4.0. Keith saw a physician because of the sudden accumulation of fluids peripherally in all his extremities.

DOCUMENTATION

If there are different techniques for the assessment of edema, it is important to document the technique used. In addition, because edema is a cyclic event, it is important to reexamine the patient at the same time of the day for every session. Comparisons with the unaffected extremity are helpful to record so that differences can be noted. The comparisons also provide information regarding when the measurements of the involved extremity resemble those of the uninvolved extremity.

If a patient is taking a diuretic, it may skew measurements and should be noted in the documentation. Sudden weight gains or losses (10 pounds or more) should be noted, as they may relate to fluid retention. Changes in treatment regimen should also be noted, as this may effect fluid retention.

Intermittent compression may be an effective tool for the patient. For sustained benefit to occur, it may be necessary for the patient to have greater access to the device, as in a rental. If the patient will be using a device, care must be taken to ensure that the patient is fully aware of the operation of the device and of potential problems that may arise. Additionally, the parameters for the device must be clearly spelled out for the patient to refer to.

Whether or not the patient uses a device outside the department, it is important to document the settings of the device. Periodic measurements should also be taken to document potential progress. The form of measurement needs to be consistent. For example, if volumetric measurements were used initially, they should be used in reevaluation of the edema.

The patient's response to the application of the device should also be recorded. Some patients may experience an increased urgency to urinate after intermittent compression. This should be documented. If fluid intake and output are monitored by the nursing staff, plans should include the measurement of the urine produced following intermittent compression.

Select two of the "patients" that you applied modalities to during the laboratory exercise, and write a progress note that includes each patient's subjective complaints, the objective information that you recorded, the physical agent that was applied, and the manner of application, the response to the applied physical agent, and your assessment.

LABORATORY QUESTIONS

1. What would be the rationale for marking off the bicepital crease as a starting point for measurement of the upper extremity?

2. What potential reasons would there be for using a vinyl tape measure?

3. What would the potential reason be for differences in the measurements that you took and that another classmate recorded?

4. If you did note differences, how would you address this in the future, or what does this mean to you?

5. Why would the time of day make any difference in the recording of edema measurements?

6. What information did the tape measure provide that the volumeter did not provide?

7. What information did the volumeter provide that the tape measure did not provide?

8. Was there any difference in the volumeter readings for the warm water versus the cold water? If yes, why? If no, why not?

9. What did your patient report to you when the intermittent compression device was operating?

10. Were there any differences between the pre-treatment and post-treatment measurements for the intermittent compression device? What would explain this?

11. What would be the rationale for a deflation pressure on this type of device?

12. Why were relatively low pressures used? Why wouldn't you use a pressure that more closely resembles the blood pressure of the patient?

13. What would explain the connection between urination and edema?

Modality Integration

Purpose

This laboratory has deliberately been placed last in this manual. Tools for any task are only as useful as the user can make them. In other words, you may have excellent tools, but they are useless if you do not know how to use them to accomplish some common treatment goals of:

Pain reduction
Muscle spasm reduction
Muscle strengthening
Muscle atrophy prevention
Edema reduction
Tissue healing
Relieving pressure on nerve roots to relieve paresthesias

The purpose of these exercises is to compare and contrast physical agent modalities in terms of the potential benefits that may be accomplished and the potential harm that may inadvertently be caused by their improper use.

Objectives

- To discriminate between physical agent modalities that can be used to accomplish similar treatment goals
- To develop a scenario in which more than one modality may be used to accomplish a cumulative effect
- To scrutinize common practice techniques to determine potential benefits, risks, and alternative methods for the accomplishment of therapeutic goals

LABORATORY EXERCISES

1. List all the possible physical agent modalities that could be used to reduce:
   a. Pain

b. Muscle spasm

c. Muscle weakness

d. Tissue healing time

e. Nerve root compression

f. Spasticity

g. Hypersensitivity

h. Edema

i. Acute inflammation

j. Chronic inflammation

k. Hematoma

2. List all the possible physical agent modalities that could be used to increase:
   a. Motor control

   b. Muscle strength

   c. Range of motion (ROM) (stretching)

   d. Muscle function

3. Which of the modalities that you mentioned in 1 and 2 would be contraindicated if the patient was pregnant: first trimester, second trimester, and third trimester?

4. Your patient has been diagnosed as having an acute cervical strain. The patient complains of pain, decreased ROM, muscle guarding, and tingling in the fingers of her right hand. What modalities could you potentially combine to treat this patient and accomplish your goals?

    a. Would ice or heat be indicated? Why?

    b. Would there be a time when either would be appropriate? If yes, when?

5. On consultation with a senior therapist, traction, ultrasound, and moist heat have been recommended to treat this patient.
    a. Which of the suggestions would you take?

    b. How would you sequence them? Why?

    c. What position would be most appropriate for this patient? Why?

6. Patient education is an important part of any therapeutic intervention.
    a. What things must you keep in mind for the patient presented in 4?

b. What behaviors do you want to be sure to warn this patient against?

7. If after applying all of the suggested modalities, the patient complained of a deep aching sensation.
   a. What would this be indicative of?

   b. How would you protect against this in the future?

8. If after treatment with the traction, muscle guarding was no longer apparent and the pain was reduced to a more tolerable level, would you proceed with ultrasound to the area as previously planned? Why or why not? (Both are possible!)

9. If after ultrasound, the patient reported that there was no paresthesia present, would you apply traction? Why or why not?

10. If after treatment (using any or all of the modalities mentioned), your patient reported that he or she now had a throbbing headache, what would this be indicative of?

11. James is a 52-year-old man who played rugby with college friends over the weekend. He has had his right knee replaced, his left ankle fused, his right hip pinned, and his rotator cuff repaired a total of two times. James does not seem to ever experience pain until real physical damage has occurred. He has been referred to the physical therapy department for the treatment of an acute episode of torticollis that is producing marked spasm in the right SCM. Once again, James reports no pain. He has commented that he actually has no sensation on the right SCM, it just "feels hard" when he touches it.

    A senior therapist in the department has recommended that you use heat and stretching to treat the torticollis. What are your plans, and how would you explain them to James and to the observing student?

12. Steve is an architect who has been referred to the physical therapy department for the relief of pain and muscle spasm in his lower back. He has difficulty maintaining an upright posture and has been told that he has a "lateral shift." On examination, Steve has weak abdominal muscles and paraspinal muscle guarding in the lumbar and thoracic spinal musculature. He complains of pain down the right leg into his ankle and difficulty with getting up from a supine position. What physical agent could be used? State the goal, the parameters to accomplish the goal, and the sequence if you suggest more than one modality.

13. You are filling in at a local outpatient therapy clinic. On reading the patient notes, you discover that all the patients you are expected to see are to receive hot packs, ultrasound, and massage in addition to joint mobilization, therapeutic exercise, and ice. How would you proceed in that setting under those circumstances?

14. After a biomedical engineering check of the ultrasound units in the clinic, it is determined that the ultrasound unit is no longer producing a therapeutic effect. You recall using it yesterday and having patients report that they felt better when you were finished. What could potentially cause them to feel better? How would you be able to prevent yourself from using an ultrasound that wasn't working again in the future?

15. A colleague read a case study by a therapist who indicated that ultrasound gel is most effective when it is cold. What are your thoughts about this? What are your thoughts about the use of ultrasound preceded or followed by ice? What additional information would you need to have in order to be able to fully address this topic?

16. A student had just finished applying ultrasound to stretch a muscle. This student is about to apply a moist heat pack to the area before beginning the stretching. What are your thoughts about this sequence? What would you do and why?

17. You are observing a treatment in which electrodes are applied to a patient's elbow and the therapist appears to be performing transverse friction massage to the lateral epicondyle. What are your thoughts about this treatment approach? What is the potential rationale for the electrical stimulation? What would the parameters need to be for this to potentially benefit the patient? If you were then asked to apply ice while the electrical stimulation continued, in your opinion would this be a good idea or a poor idea?